LIVING WITH OUR HYPERACTIVE CHILDREN

LIVING WITH OUR HYPERACTIVE CHILDREN

Edited by
Marvin L. Bittinger

Foreword by
John F. Zimmer, M.D.
Pediatrician

BPS Books, Inc.
Two Continents Publishing Group, Ltd.

Library of Congress Cataloging in Publication Data
Main entry under title:

Living with our hyperactive children.

1. Hyperactive children–Biography. 2. Psychology, Religious. I. Bittinger, Marvin L.
RJ506.H9L58 618.9'28'58 76-56681
ISBN 0-8467-0275-4

Joshua copyright info
EVERYBODY HAS A HISTORY

From Mister Rogers Record
Come On and Wake Up!

Printed in the United States of America
Two Continents Publishing Group, Ltd.
30 East 42nd Street
New York, NY 10017
and BPS Books, Inc.

Each of the personal histories in this book are true. All names have been changed.

Dedicated to all parents of children
with special problems.

CONTENTS

PUBLISHER'S NOTE

There are distinct writing styles and methods of expression in each section of this book, and an effort has been made to preserve this personal approach—for this is a very personal book. Human emotions and personal feelings come from the individual, not from an editor's pencil, and this is why the parents who wrote these stories were willing to make their contributions. We hope that this will make the book mean that much more to the reader, as it does to these very special people who wrote it.

INTRODUCTION

I was a hyperactive child. Now I am a pediatrician in private practice. I was asked by the author to share some of my thoughts about hyperactive children, from both a personal standpoint as a hyperactive child and a professional standpoint as a practicing pediatrician.

My cause for having minimal brain dysfunction (a synonym for hyperactivity) was starting life too early, as a three-pound, seven-month-old premature baby. I was a sickly infant, cared-for by a loving mother who fed me with a medicine dropper and kept my crib by the kitchen stove. I have been told about my busy impulsive behavior during my early, pre-memory stage of life. I needed to be constantly eating a cookie or a cracker in order to hold still long enough to have my picture taken. In the early movies of my first steps, taken by my father, I always seem to be running off somewhere. I used to run outside every time a train whistle blew to see it pass by three blocks away. I was a "biter." Once I bit my puppy after he bit me (we were both teething at the time). I also bit people. Each time one of my former neighbors sees my mother she still asks if her son bites. My favorite pastime was unrolling toilet paper. Upon entering first grade, I found it easier to spell backwards than forwards. My mother finally taught me to spell forwards, but only after a solid year of working with me on the problem. Television was not invented then, so little did we know that I could have been groomed to be a Professor Backwards (a TV personality in the fifties who could write words backwards). At my birthday party, age eight, I stuck my paper napkin into a burning candle to see what would happen. My father had to stomp out the fire, as I stood paralyzed, holding the burning torch. When asked why, I really had to say "I don't know." I just felt the urge, even though I knew in my own mind what would happen. To this day, I still don't know why I did that.

All through school, it took me an hour to do a 15-minute lesson because I could not concentrate and would daydream. I missed a lot of playing time because of this problem. Often I would arise at 5:30 a.m. and ride my bicycle for two hours before leaving for school, I was clumsy while playing at games on the recess ground, so consequently, I was the last person chosen for a team. School tests became a problem when I read the wrong words into the questions. I scored poorly on my college entrance exam, although I made National Honor Society all but three six-week periods during high school. The school principal told my mother I wasn't college material. Luckily, she didn't tell me until I had graduated from medical school. My first semester on a college campus I was on probation and I finished the first year on condition that I improve my grade-point average the next year. Then, I seemed to gel at age eighteen, and, although I was told by the medical admissions board my junior year of college that I didn't have a "Chinaman's chance in hell" of being accepted, I made the dean's list in my senior year and was accepted to medical school that following summer. I graduated in the upper half of my medical school class; and in 1970 I successfully passed my American Academy of Pediatrics boards. Incidentally, the oral tests were easier for me than the written tests, I still am not a speed reader, and I find taped lessons and lectures easier to understand than written matter. Some people now call me a successful pediatrician.*

Now that I have shared my personal involvement in the hyperactive syndrome, let me share some insights revealed to me during my practice of pediatrics.

What is a child? No two people view this question alike, I think the best way I know to answer this most fundamental question is to state what a child is *not.* (My use of the pronoun

*Author's Comment: Parents of hyperactive children hold him in especially high regard.

"he" is not intended to be sexist, though hyperactivity is seen far more often in boys than in girls by a ratio of 7:1.) A child is not a little adult and, therefore, doesn't look, think, feel, or act in an adult manner. He is not very logical, but lives much of his existence in a play world where the real and the unreal are often intertwined to the point of losing their distinctness. Often discipline and/or the attention to stick to a task is lacking. Instead of suppressing "lousy" feelings children more often express them to the point of irritating other people. People are often seen as they really are, not as they pretend to be. Tact is lacking so feelings are expressed exactly as they are perceived. There is no censorship of words; expression is exactly what comes to mind. If someone has a big nose, a child tells him so. Frustration of desires is usually expressed immediately. Daily tasks are sometimes forgotten because something needs to be done in a hurry so he can go on with life. Therefore, there are messes made and objects destroyed in the process. Limits, although they give a feeling of security, are tested time and time again to see if one can bend the rules. When a limit fails, the fact that the child has to control himself, but doesn't know how, increases his anxiety.

If this constitutes a "normal child," then what makes a child hyperactive? The answer is that hyperactive children do all the things normal children do only more often and/or more intensively. Perception of increased activity is in the eye of the beholder and depends on his tolerance level. There are some basic inherited personality types, from docile, easy-to-please, passive, easily channeled behavior (often seen in small girls) to the active, hard-to-please, aggressive, search-and-destroy behavior (often seen in boys). Nonetheless, there are some medical norms about children, and deviation to the extremes of behavior serves as a red flag warning of future problems. Medical literature lists the following as the most likely behaviors associated with the hyperactive syndrome: short attention span, distractibility, impulsiveness, overactiveness, clumsiness, right-left confusion, specific learning problems (writing, spelling, reading, word confusion, math, and so on), low activity (daydreaming or spending too long at a task—perseveration) and poor sleeping habits. Essentially, the hyperactive child is an exaggerated normal child.

The first step in recognizing a hyperactive child is to ask one's self, "Does a problem exist with my child?" The realistic answer to this question is the first step toward the solution. People have to be realists and see that a problem exists before they can be open to working toward a solution. Why do parents have a difficult time facing this question? Ego gets in the way; and, as the holy scriptures have recorded, in the three thousand years of human existence man has wanted to be independent and not rely on God and other men's help in solving his problems. Mothers, therefore, blame themselves instead of seeking solutions: fathers, whom scriptures command to control and lead their families, deny the problem, and if it doesn't disappear they blame everyone or anyone including their wives, rather than seeking help by admitting the problems are too big for them to solve. This is because we men have been taught since we were children that it is a sign of non-manliness to ask for help and admit some of our weaknesses to another person. Yet it is in sharing these weaknesses (problems) that cures (solutions) take place.

Now the question: How do we care for the hyperactive child? First of all, parents must see that attitudes are correct between family members. Of primary importance is the father and mother relationship as husband and wife. Do their actions reveal loving acceptance of one another? If they do not, how can they realistically show acceptance toward children, especially if one child is a problem child? Nonacceptance by parents causes anxiety in healthy children, and more so in impulsive, hyperactive children. This is not to deny that divorced parents can't help a hyperactive child, but they must be mature enough to accept the estranged spouse, even if it is not loving acceptance. Otherwise no consistent, unified example can be given the child to teach him to grow towards adult maturity.

We who have the responsibility of helping families with the hyperactive syndrome must also work through the same priorities. We need to be free enough to tell families "I don't know" instead of making educated guesses and passing them off as the only answer. Our biggest tool for helping is the will to listen and to try to share the family's burden to make their load lighter. Otherwise we become cynical about our feelings and then try to get rid of these problem families as quickly as possible with the least amount of vested time. Here I am speaking not only of the medical profession but of psychologists, social workers, teachers, special educators, and government workers. They deny the truth and perceive the nonexistence of a problem as truth.

Many well-meaning people have advanced many theories as solutions to the problem of hyperactivity—such as megavitamins or diet manipulation. Most of these theories have suffered from the inability of other medical people to duplicate the results. These, in my experience, have proved useless, except that there does seem to be some success when a child has low blood sugar. This type of problem has been solved in about half the cases of frequent, small protein-feedings. *Some medications have also proved helpful in helping increase the child's awareness and attention span. These drugs do nothing to control behavior in themselves or make a child good or bad; they are not a substitute for loving acceptance, special methods teaching, firm limits and direction, one-on-one attention, and parent-parent, parent-teacher, and parent-doctor doctor communications in a truthful, trustful relationship.* The five most useful drugs I have found are the following, in order of effectiveness: Ritalin® (a stimulant), Cylert® (a stimulant), Dexadrine® (a stimulant), Mellaril® (a tranquilizer and stimulant), and Dilantin® (a seizure medication-anticonvulsant). Coffee (a stimulant), without sugar, also has helped, but not caffeine tablets.

Why are we seeing more of the MBD (Minimal brain dysfunction), or hyperactive behavior, today? Is it because we place too many demands on the child to perform without allowing him the freedom to not perform sometimes? Is life becoming too complicated? Is the child's worth only what he becomes in an adult's eye and not who he sees himself to be? I leave you with these questions to answer in your own hearts and minds.

Why are we critical, conditional lovers? The only thing that can change a person's life and attitudes is unconditional love. God, who is both perfect Father and Mother, is waiting to teach us how, through his family of mankind. As you read through these stories that people have cared to share on paper, I hope you get the help and encouragement you need for the hyperactive child in your life.

John F. Zimmer, M.D.
Pediatrician

FOREWORD

Many books have been written by child psychologists and other professional people concerning the hyperactive child. These books tend to take a view from the outside telling parents what to do. None of these books look at the problem from the inside, exploring the parents' feelings and how they have coped with the hyperactive child. We do not attempt to give professional opinions as if we were doctors or psychologists, but nevertheless we have tried to provide a "professionally" written account, in straightforward terms, of the problems encountered through the parents' eyes. The core of this book is seven stories about hyperactive children written by their parents in conjunction with the editor. One of these stories is about the editor's child. There is no better method for parents of hyperactive chldren to know that their special agony is understood by others than to read others' experiences, to know those who have shared the experiences and in some way have learned to cope — even to constructively improve their situation where medical people could not hope to assist.

As one reads the stories, a common thread will emerge; and it is this common thread that we hope will help and comfort other parents in the situation. The names of the parents, except that of the editor, have been changed at their request; all names of the children have been changed.

WHAT IS A *HYPERACTIVE* CHILD?

It is very difficult to stereotype hyperactivity. It is more a cluster of symptoms than any one problem: delay in development, poor coordination, social difficulties, poor attention span, extreme physical activity, or some brain damage. If there is one single way of describing the physical basis of hyperactivity, it is that some amount of neurological impairment exists, but the important thing to keep in mind is that this ranges along a continuum from minimal to moderate. There are hyperactive children who are in constant motion, always physically active. This is the way the syndrome is demonstrated by them, but this may not be the case for all hyperactive children. Some hyperactive children are actually very docile. If there is one overt manifestation of hyperactivity it is poor attention span (attention disorder), but this type of child need *not* be physically active. A hyperactive child can be very passive, not playing with anything for very long, or simply not listening. It is typical of hyperactive children not to screen out stimuli. They respond to everything in their environment. Their tracking system has not matured. They are like two-year olds, always distracted by visual and auditory stimuli yet not sticking with any one stimulus very long. The intellectual capability of the hyperactive child can range from low to very high.

In summary, hyperactivity is a cluster of symptoms, not all of which occur in every hyperactive child. The predominate symptoms can be generalized as neurological impairment and attention disorder.

WRITING THE BOOK

Some comments about how the writing took place may be helpful before you start reading. Each of the people worked independently of the others, following a general outline provided by the editor. You will find the stories differing in many ways; one may be more analytical, another more emotional, and another more clinical. Some wrote in a very terse style, while others were more detailed. From a personal standpoint, I felt quite comfortable editing the stories of others, but writing my own was the most painful. It is so hard to sort out one's true feelings. Was my feeling of anger true and deep, or was it just a temporary state of emotion, that I could shrug off in time? To summarize, while some of the stories may seem more from the heart than others, let me assure you that *all* of them came from the hearts of these parents, and I want to express my deep appreciation to them for pouring out their souls in this writing.

One final note of caution which is not meant to be negative, just honest. Feel assured that this book is not proposing final and absolute answers to this problem. We as parents of hyperactive children are so desperate for help that we become easy prey to gimmicks and hopeful promises regarding our problems. Approach any solution, given in this book or any other, with awareness and caution. Nevertheless, I am almost certain that you will find some helpful suggestions in these pages (I know I did). The biggest challenge of all may be to carry them out.

Best wishes to you!
MLB

JOSHUA

While some of these stories do not delve into personal feelings, Joshua's mother is able to portray the emotions of her family vividly, to show there is nothing unusual about negative feelings that often develop when hope seems slim—as long as the reader sees that hope is a very important part of dealing with such a child. Joshua was probably the opposite of what would normally be thought to be a "hyperactive child." He was very slow in accomplishing any kind of physical activity. He sat without movement for much of his early life. Today, he is certainly active and is seen as a hyperactive child. Joshua remains the only child in his family, for his parents see great advantages to one child, who requires such an extreme amount of time.

I hated today

I hated the clinical neurologist
who made me wait with my child
for forty-five minutes in a waiting room
that had nothing for a child to touch

except

a bell

to which
a cranky old receptionist

blurted, "Don't play with that,"
and in a cold clipped tone
she added, to me,

"Could you kindly take that bell from your child
and put it back on the counter?"

I hated, after forty-five minutes of waiting,

being brought into a small examining room,
with nothing to do but wait
and not touch all of the doctor's untouchables.

And I hated my answers to the doctor's questions.
I didn't like being reminded why I was there,
that my child was different.

And after a few questions and some instructions
to get him undressed,
I hated being left without explanation
for another half-hour wait.

And I hated myself for not remembering
to bring toys and crayons and books
for all that waiting.

After the examination comes the consultation.
"How did it happen?"
And asking the same old questions of a new doctor
And asking myself, "Why my child?"
And hating that all the answers and
information in the world won't change
anything for my child.

And why do doctors give their conferences with your child there?
I hate that when a child is tired and cross
and old enough to understand

your talking about what's wrong with him
instead of what's right with him...

And then some tests were prescribed;
"The child needs to be sedated because
he can't sit still," I heard.

I hated the receptionist again,
because she didn't understand about children
and I hated that my child didn't understand about sedation
and refused the syrupy liquid,
spitting it back at the receptionist.

I hated the lonely feeling
waiting in the crowded laboratory reception room
while a small child went in for full skull Xrays.

And I hated again, while I waited
and they measured his brain waves

And then
"Please wait to see if the doctor wants to see you"
and after twenty minutes of waiting being old
"No, wait until Monday and the doctor will call you."

And all of that waiting and hating—was just routine.

He is a beautiful child, blond hair, a big smile
and eyes that sometimes sparkle...but
this day he walked funny. The sedative upset
his equilibrium and his hair still had white
paste in it from the EEG. Earlier in the day
he asked for ice cream and I said
"Yes—when we are finished."

Inside the ice cream parlor I heard a voice ask,
"What's the matter with him, Mommy?"
and I saw a finger pointing at my child.
In a loud voice the mother responded,
"Oh, him, can't you see, he is retarded?"

And I hated that mother
And I hated her child
And I hated all my hating.

And underneath all the hating

I hurt.

HISTORY OF CHILD

It's hard to begin writing Joshua's story. His story is one of events, feelings, attitudes, frustrations, hopes and dreams. Joshua was a planned child. He was wanted by his mother and father.

Joshua's history began generations before he was born. It began with me, his mother, and how I was raised, and it began with his dad and how he was raised. I came from a generation of mothers who sacrificed their lives for their children. I can remember being eight years old and overhearing Grandma yelling at my mother, "Is this all I get from you, after sacrificing my life for you kids?" My mother never said that to me. She didn't have to. I could see it in how she lived her life. Her first marriage left her widowed with three small children. I was five years old and my sisters were six and eight. Two things stand out in my memory. One is that it is my belief that, when my mother remarried, it was more for my sister and me than it was for her. Her children needed a father. The other evidence of sacrifice was that Mom took the modest amount of money that came from Dad's estate and saved it for the future education of my sister and me. She didn't have much for herself in those days, and she was responsible for three. Coming from such a background, it's not surprising than one of the qualities I was looking for in a marriage partner was a man who would make a good father for my children.

I was twenty-six when I married David. I loved him, he loved me and he liked children.

David was raised by his mother. His father died of cancer shortly after David was born. He had an older brother and sister. David's mother worked. She was a nurse and often worked seven days a week. David spent many hours with neighborhood families. He adopted them and they adopted him. These were lasting relationships, and part of the family background that David brought to our marriage.

From the time of our marriage to the time of Joshua's birth, four years had passed. David had spent three of them in graduate school and a year after that working for a large corporation. I had worked during these four years and quit my job only weeks before Joshua was due to be born. Those were busy weeks. I went to garage and rummage sales, and with David refinished baby furniture and read about how babies are born. David and I did a lot of reading together. We made decisions on such things as Pampers versus diapers and breast versus bottle. Around the fifth month of pregnancy my obstetrician mentioned that the baby was in a breech position. Three months later during my monthly checkup, the doctor attempted, in what seemed to me like a token gesture, to turn the baby. Nothing happened.

My pregnancy was relatively uneventful. The first six weeks were the most difficult. I was extremely tired, and my stomach was weak at inopportune moments, like driving home from work in rush hour traffic. For the most part it was a quiet pregnancy. I kept looking forward to feeling the baby move around inside of me; I had read that it would happen and people kept asking, "Do you feel anything yet?" I didn't. Uterine movement was minimal and I came to consider this normal for a breech birth.

After becoming pregnant I started reading about prenatal development and care, labor and childbirth. David and I decided we wanted to try natural childbirth, and we traveled sixty miles for instructions. We were probably a typical couple, eager to do everything right for our first baby.

The first thought of abnormality and childbirth was a fleeting, but significant, one. The hospital where our baby was to be delivered allows fathers to be present during delivery, provided the parents have taken the baby classes given by the hospital and the delivery requires no surgical procedures. The classes were taught by a personable and knowledgeable nurse. It was the third week of class and in her attempt to calm our prenatal anxieties she told us not to worry about childbirth, that 98 percent of all births were normal children. I remember counting about forty people sitting in the room, mostly couples, and whispering to David, "Well, that must mean one of us sitting here isn't going to have a normal baby." There was another statistic floating around in my head at that time: it was under the category of breech births. I couldn't remember the specifics, but I knew the chances for difficulties were greatly increased for babies in that position.

I thought I was ready for labor; I knew what was going to happen; I had done well with my Lamaze instruction and David and I continued to practice relaxation and breathing on a regular basis. We had learned about the use of anesthetics in delivery and had made a decision to breast feed. The crib was painted and my suitcase was packed. I was ready and I was scared. Labor, enemas, delivery episiotomy, and pain threshold, were all words that could activate my scared feelings.

Well, labor and delivery didn't happen like the books or the nurse said. The doctor had said little. Only the Lamaze instructor talked about abnormal births, but I must not have been listening, because I wanted to have a normal labor and delivery just like everyone else. I was awakened out of a sleep with my first labor pains. I got out the stop watch and began timing my contractions. They were irregular and they hurt, and I was unable to control them with the first and second stages of breathing, which I had so carefully practiced the weeks before. (The third stage of breathing was designed for the last stages of labor.) This worried me. I waited until 7 a.m. and called my obstetrician. He dismissed my symptoms as false labor on the grounds that my contractions were not regular. With that information David left for work and I stayed home. Between contractions, I paced the floor like an expectant father, wondering why false labor was so painful to me, and then scared myself by thinking, "If this is false labor, what will the real thing be like?" Feeling like a failure, I called David home; he called our Lamaze instructor and she advised us to get to the doctor immediately. She reported that irregular contractions were false symptoms for a normally positioned child, but it was her experience that this was typical labor for breech babies.

The doctor agreed to see me in his office, found me dilated to eight centimeters (ten is delivery), and left an office full of waiting patients while he rushed to meet us at the hospital. Xrays and hard contractions allowed the doctor to continue with our decision for me to have my baby naturally. Three hours later, still dilated at eight, the decision was changed to Cesarean section delivery. There was a two-hour delay waiting for a surgery room to become available. David was supportive during the long wait for delivery, and having him with me was what I needed to keep myself in control of the contractions and continue with the special breathing. (Lamaze breathing reportedly allows for more oxygen to the baby during the time of contractions.) At 7 p.m. I had a spinal anesthetic and was awake for the birth. Joshua weighed eight pounds, seven ounces, was twenty-two inches long and in good general health. David was happy with the birth and very disappointed he was not a witness to it.

Joshua was the first child to parents who had no previous experience with babies. He was a child who was not grossly impaired. Black and white are definite, but what's gray? Joshua was born at a time in my life when I was unsure of myself. It wasn't visible on the outside. I had lived an active life. I had a graduate degree and had six years of work experience in professional positions. Inside the home I excelled in cooking and entertaining, and still I was unsure of myself. I wanted to be a good mother. There were many things about having my first baby that raised doubts in myself. I enjoyed nursing Joshua, but how did I know he was really getting enough milk? He was skinny; neither my mother nor my mother-in-law had nursed her children, and hearing a question like, "Are you sure he's getting enough to eat?" would get the conflict spinning inside of me.

I had always worked, and although it was still a possibility after the baby was born, it was in my head that good mothers stay home with their babies.

A few months after Joshua was born David changed jobs. He went from a nine-to-five corporate position, to working for a small company. A combination of the new demands of his position and David's desire to succeed in his work had him working from 9 a.m. to 7 or 8 p.m. or midnight, whatever the job required, and as many days of the week as were needed, six and on some occasions even seven. We had lived in the city for a few years, and I had worked most of that time. I didn't know many people, and had only a couple of friends. I was at home a lot, and those early days and months and years were lonely ones for me. There was a big need for emotional support, and little things like a telephone call home, taken from a busy day, would have meant a lot. But there were no calls. During the days when David did not see Joshua, I would keep him updated with the events of our days. David was always interested in Joshua, and in what and how he was doing.

The feelings that I remember the most during this time were being lonely and being scared. The best prescription would have been knowing another parent like me with whom to share concerns. I feel that most mothers who have children with special needs will need more supportive husbands, and single parents raising a special child would benefit from a supportive friend or group. As the months went into years it became apparent that David and I were not touching each other's lives as we once did—we weren't responding to each other. I became aware that I stopped reaching out. I didn't want to any more. It seemed like when I did, it was in an atmosphere of tension and frustration. These were problems of the marriage that Joshua had nothing to do with.

From Mister Rogers Record,
Come On and Wake Up!

EVERYBODY HAS A HISTORY

You were born a baby and then you grew,
And you grew and you grew and you grew,
And you grew.
And now you can do what a baby couldn't do,
Your story is your history.

Everybody has a history
Everybody has a name
Everybody has a story
No one's story is exactly the same,
As anyone else's.

I was born a baby and then I grew,
And I grew and I grew and I grew and I grew.
And now I can do what a baby couldn't do.
My story is my history.
My story is my history.

HOW I FOUND ABOUT THE DISABILITY

Hey Lady, You have a child—be happy
He has two arms, two legs, eight fingers, two thumbs
and ten toes — be happy
And I know someone who would trade you
for his blond hair and blue eyes — be happy

Hey Lady, nothing's wrong with your kid,
that he doesn't walk?
I have a neighbor who's kid didn't walk
until he was four—be happy

Look Lady, if your pediatrician didn't tell you to worry
don't worry — be happy

I can't see a thing wrong with your kid—
Mine can always find someone who can do something better
than him. Don't worry.
Hey Lady, don't worry—
it's just a delay

Damn it,
I'm worried —
about my baby and
about what's wrong with me
that I need to have something
wrong with my child
and worry if
there's nothing to worry about
and nothing's wrong.

What I think of first is not how I found out about Joshua's disability, but how I didn't. Joshua is a healthy child. He never visited the pediatrician for anything other than routine developmental office visits. He's never missed a day of school due to illness. By the end of his first year I became aware that these routine appointments with the pediatrician were making me anxious. It seemed as if I could not answer yes to the doctor's inquiries on Joshua's motor development until two to four appointments after they were first asked. I had questions, too, like why was Joshua eating so much and not gaining much weight? His stomach was bloated and grotesque in size and the doctor instructed me to let him eat as much as he wanted. "He knows when to stop," but that child never stopped. Joshua ate frantically and in volume ate more than me. He stopped eating only when I stopped feeding him. He never left any food on his plate. Other mothers reassured me that all babies' stomachs are big. I'd never been a mother before, and I had no means of comparison. I only knew that I felt anxious about it. It was the summer before Joshua's first birthday. David, who shared my questions and had some of his own, wasn't satisfied with the answers I would bring home from the pediatrician. David would ask me questions that I didn't want to hear. I would get defensive, wanting to believe the doctor, that his food intake was OK, but I was faced with the fact that something was wrong every time there was a meal. A pound of peanut butter and a two-pound container of cottage cheese were among snacking foods for Joshua during a one-week period. He had other eating habits that seemed odd as he grew older. I would be preparing a stew and he would grab large pieces of raw onions and potatoes and eat them like raisins if not stopped. (Much later two hypotheses were suggested about the origin of Joshua's eating habits. First, his sensory feedback system was not developing and he never had the feeling of fullness or discomfort when he ate. His stomach muscles, being soft and flaccid, had no resistance to food and liquid as he ate. Second, because he was slow in gaining control over his body, he relied on his oral needs for self-satisfaction.) In hindsight, I should have trusted my feelings and been more sure that something was wrong. After a visit with the pediatrician I was sure the doctor thought I was a pushy, middle-class Jewish mother who was uptight because her first-born son wasn't the first to walk and talk. I knew the stereotype, and I knew that that was not me. One of the important lessons David and I learned was to think through problems on our own. We slowly evolved to a point where we would listen to the professionals, listen to our own feelings, be aware of our child and the situation, and synthesize all three.

There is a saying that sticks out in my head about "even your best friends won't tell you." One was Jean, a woman who lived in my parents' home town. She is a PhD., and among her professional responsibilities as directing a pre-Head Start program, working with pregnant mothers, newborns, and children up to age three. She had had experience with hundreds of babies and was concerned that something was wrong with my baby. She shared her concern only after we began having Joshua tested. My other friend was a psychiatrist. Don and I had worked together at a mental health center and remained friends and colleagues after I'd left the center. He'd had some experience with children and had raised three of his own. Again, it was only after I began to verbalize my concern about Joshua that he reported he had some concerns about the child and eventually would have said something to me about it. Later I went back and asked Jean and Don what it was that made them question Joshua's development. They both felt that he lacked responsiveness to his environment. He stared a lot and often wore a blank expression.

I used to ask myself why I was later than David and my friends in recognizing Joshua's problem. In part it was my lack of experience with babies, and in part it was an unconscious unwillingness to deal with the anger, fear, guilt, and realities that recognition would bring.

Ironically, there were a couple of things that I did early in Joshua's life that may have delayed my identification of his problem. By my third month of pregnancy I began to feel good; terrific, in fact. I began exercising, taking long walks, and swimming whenever I could. I had a quick recovery from a Cesarean section birth. After Joshua was born I continued with postnatal exercises and when he was three weeks old I started him on Bonnie Pruden exercises, *How to Keep Your Child Fit From Birth To Six*. I thought the program was excellent and easy to follow. I would work with him once or twice a day, an opportunity that was made easier for me because Joshua was my first child and I wasn't working. What I found was that he did not progress as quickly as Bonnie Pruden's program suggested. Joshua did fine on the exercises where I did all the muscle manipulations, but he became fussy and uncooperative during the exercises requiring him to help in some muscular movements. He was about nine months old when we began doing the exercises that were scheduled for six-month-old babies. We had fallen three months behind. This group of exercises included upper body and back lifts and prone and supine leg lifts. It became evident that Joshua didn't like any exercises where a part of his body was not supported by a chair, the floor, or me. I found our exercises were becoming a chore, something I felt we should be doing. I didn't look anything like the smiling mother in the book and Joshua looked nothing like the baby Rene in the illustrations. The book illustrated a mother working with her laughing baby, while Joshua cried because of what I did to him. I couldn't understand what I was doing wrong. I'd go back and reread the exercises, making sure I was executing them correctly. There were too many tears and too many fears, and finally we stopped. What I didn't know then was that Joshua had problems with motor and muscle activity. The exercises helped develop muscles that Joshua wasn't developing on his own and at the same time delayed recognition of the problem. I must have wondered a hundred times, How much further along would Joshua be if I hadn't quit? Vivian, the first professional to evaluate Joshua, asked, "I wonder how much further behind he would be if you hadn't worked so diligently with him during those first nine months?" I stopped because Joshua's response to activity made it an unhappy experience for both of us. This was the first reminder of the constant interplay between physical (and much later, intellectual) and emotional growth.

On the subject of Jolly Jumpers, Bonnie Pruden writes one short chapter and says, "The best piece of baby apparatus I have ever seen is the Jolly Jumper." Joshua had received a super deluxe model for a baby gift. I had seen my neighbor's baby girl spend joyous moments laughing and pleasing herself as she moved about in hers. They came highly recommended, guaranteed to bring giggles and joy. Jolly Jumpers were not jolly for Joshua. He just hung there limp and unresponsive to my gestures and proddings. If left on his own he cried. I didn't have a jolly baby and I didn't know why.

When Joshua was six months old I enrolled him in a Tiny Tots gym and swim class. He was the youngest baby in the class and we were in luck because the teacher was doing exercises we had already practiced. This was also his introduction to swimming, an activity that today Joshua has begun to master.

Joshua's development progressed slowly, but always progressed. He was holding his head up at four months, sitting at seven months, crawling around at nine months, and gave us his first unsteady walking steps at eighteen months. He was not an active child. He didn't crawl very much, even after he learned how; he was content to sit in one place. (This was an early clue to David.)

Other mothers complained that their kids were into everything and said how lucky I was with Joshua. By this time I was into what I've labeled the cooperative era of my life. I was into playgroup, food, and baby-sitting cooperatives. Playgroup was filled with mothers trying to provide all of the right experiences for their children. Their main purpose for getting together was to be involved in a part of their children's play experiences. I observed other mothers enjoying the playground experience, sharing stories about all the cute things their children were doing, and watching their children progress. For me it was the painful awareness that something was wrong. At playgroup you worked one morning and got one morning off. On mornings when I worked, when I would move away from Joshua he would cry, and I didn't understand why. He was that way wherever we went. It took eight months for him to adjust to the group on mornings I worked. I hated those mornings, with Joshua crying and the slow painful awareness that my child was different from those other children. Even at home, if I walked out of a room, Joshua would sit there and cry until I came back into sight. Slowly I was coming to grips with the fact that something wasn't right. (In spite of the difficulties, I was glad I joined the playgroup. It forced me to see Joshua in comparison to a lot of other children his own age — and to distinguish between individual differences and gross deviation.)

Getting no support from our pediatrician, who had a wait-and-see attitude, David and I decided that if we were still concerned when Joshua was two years old we would take him for testing. At age two Joshua was still walking like a beginner, and he cried if we were outside in tall grass or ivy that was around the house. He would refuse to lift his legs. He'd be upset and we were upset. What we didn't know was that he couldn't lift his legs, that he hadn't yet developed the physical apparatus to do what we thought came naturally for children.

While David was first aware of slow motor development, I was more aware of Joshua's delay in language. As an infant he babbled a lot, and we thought he would be an early talker. I talked to him a lot and I used to think he was babbling back sentences, but he never progressed from there. He was two years old before he could repeat or imitate sounds. At twenty-seven months he was saying simple words like *bye, Mama,* and *shoes.* My mother tried to reassure me by telling me she had heard that Einstein didn't talk until he was four years old. There were other well-meaning comments passed along about other famous people who didn't walk until some late age. I can remember wondering what it is about me that is creating this problem that doesn't exist.

The behavior that made me the most unsure of myself was Joshua's tantrums. When they began, somewhere in his second year, I was bewildered as to what triggered them off. They went like this: Joshua would cry and then hold his breath until his face turned blue. His body and appendages would stiffen and then he would fall like a board. There were two things to deal with here. First, I was concerned for Joshua's safety. He would have these tantrums on the stairs or while climbing onto something, and falling usually meant potential danger. Second, I grew short on tolerance for the tantrum behavior and long on frustration with my continued inability to resolve the problem. I was able to deal with the first; a watchful eye and quick maneuvers kept Joshua safe. I never solved the second problem. By the summer before his second birthday he was having eighteen to twenty tantrums a day. This went on for three or four months before they slowly began to taper off in number. By the end of the summer I understood what was causing the tantrums — some frustrating factor in his environment. Sometimes it was Mother, sometimes it was his inability to get a block that dropped out of his reach. Whatever it was, at first I was the only one Joshua tantrumed for, and until David had experienced one I always thought he felt I was exaggerating. He told people that Joshua was an easy baby to care for. The reality was that David didn't know. He wasn't there. I began to doubt myself and my abilities to be the mother I wanted to be. I didn't know what to do with all of these months of crying, and every tantrum triggered a voice in my head saying, "What's the matter with you"?

What kept me going during that time was my friend, Don, who believed in me while I was doubting myself. If I would bitch and complain about the mothers at playgroup, he would say "It's OK to be scared," putting me in touch with my real feelings. And if on a bad day I would sometimes say, "I'm not even sure if I love that kid," he didn't think I was a bad person. On those days that I couldn't love my child, Don's confidence in me kept me from hating myself.

In July 1972 I was reading the current issue of *Parents Magazine*. Joshua was twenty-two months old then. There was an article on minimal brain dysfunction in children. When I got to the part describing the symptoms I was readily aware that they were describing Joshua. The article mentioned Dr. Kephart and a university, less than one hundred miles from our home, where they were working with these children. That was the catalyst that put our search for information about Joshua into action. I gave the article to David to read that night and we made a rare quick decision to call Dr. Kephart the next day. Five telephone calls later I learned that Dr. Kephart was no longer at the university, but the achievement center would send out an application for testing and diagnosis. In November 1972 I began writing answers to a preliminary information form and sixteen pages later returned it to the Special Education Department at the achievement center. In February 1973 we took Joshua to the achievement center at Purdue for his first evaluation. He was twenty-nine months old.

That Joshua had a problem in development was confirmed that day. The details will be described later. I asked the therapist what we could expect in terms of Joshua's future. What can I fear and what can I hope or dream? "The worst thing that can happen is that you will have to institutionalize your child one day and the best thing is that he will be able to take care of himself and live and work in society." Then he could be normal," I added. "No, not in the sense like you and me," she said.

It had been a long day. It began at 6 a.m. with an hour and a half drive to the evaluation center. Testing included observation of Joshua (by staff members with a variety of specialties) while he was alone and while he was interacting with his parents. The evaluation ended with parent conferences. We came with a lot of questions and left with few answers, but what we did leave with was a lot of instructions for things to do for Joshua. I remember riding home in the car and feeling a sense of relief, and resolved that if anyone could do something for that child, I could.

FEELING GOOD and FEELING BAD in OUR FAMILY

My husband is in business and a few months ago
he went into business for himelf.
On good days he says, "I'm self-employed."
On bad days he says, "I'm unemployed."

When I'm feeling good it doesn't matter what
I'm doing:
running errands
folding laundry
pulling weeds....

When I'm feeling bad it matters what
I'm doing. I need to be doing something
important, like
teaching
reading
writing.....
To prove that I'm OK.

Some people say my son is retarded. This is
obvious in the area of feeling bad. He
refuses to learn how to feel bad.
Everyday he races with his friend on his
big wheel and everyday he reports with a
smile,
Jimmy was first today
and then I was first.

FAMILY ADJUSTMENT

The days, weeks, and months following our visit to the achievement center were busy ones. I had a job to do, a challenge to meet. The testing results noted that Joshua had problems of balance and general coordination. He was unsteady in his movements and there was a wobbliness in his trunk when he was standing still. That was why even lifting one leg was difficult, if not impossible, for Joshua at this time. They observed that considerable effort was required of him to perform even the most minimal task. Joshua lacked muscle tone. They showed us that when you squeezed him he felt rubbery. We heard the term *hypotonic.* Joshua couldn't jump or run, and they observed that his right foot did not come down to the floor when he walked.

We further learned that the information he received from his feedback system was low and consequently inadequate to support learning and development. Joshua was essentially a nonverbal child. Now there was a lot of work to be done. We received pages and pages of instructions. There were exercises to develop muscles, curiosity, and general physical competence. Activities and exercises were planned to teach Joshua to lift his legs, climb over objects, and to roll and balance. David spent his free time making equipment. I read mimeographed materials that instructed us on developmental linguistic techniques for teaching language-delayed children. I would summarize for David and we both learned new ways of talking to Joshua. The results with language were exciting. His vocabulary increased within a week. We had a much longer wait for results in other areas.

For the next seven months about 75 percent of my waking hours were devoted to working with or planning for Joshua. Bath time was water-play exercises. There were daily routines of exercises, walking up and down hills, learning to critically evaluate expectations so that Joshua knew success every day. I learned patience and control. I learned to let him struggle. If it meant five minutes for him to climb into the back seat of the car, then we took five minutes. I was a believer in early childhood intervention, and a child's future was at stake — my child's. But where did the energy to implement this total planning come from? Now I believe that giving all of my energy to Joshua was how I handled my guilt. There were always the nagging questions: How did this happen? Why did it happen? Was it labor, delivery, or some medication I'd taken? Joshua was a little more than a year old when I began psychiatric treatment. I talked about Joshua a lot, always looking for an answer, wanting to absolve myself from my own accusations. David didn't feel guilty—in my mixed-up thinking I concluded it had to be me!

While guilt seemed to be my motivating source of energy, it also served to block my anger. I never got angry, lost my temper, or raised my voice. I grew up in a family where I had never had permission to be angry. I was not in touch with my own anger, and that feeling was always a scary one to me. A cold, icy glare from my mother could send me running to my room feeling guilty for some wrongdoing. I was afraid of my mother's anger or anyone else's. As I grew older I would go to great lengths to avoid someone's angry feelings. Even today, I feel anxious when someone I care about is angry with me. (It's part of an old mixed-up thinking, that if you're angry with me, you can't love me.)

Instead of getting angry, I got headaches. They could last for two to five days. My head hurt when I walked, and I would wake from sleep with a throbbing ache. I cried a lot too in those days, and crying always left me with swollen eyes, a red nose, and an aching head. I was not aware of my anger—it was masked with feeling hurt. In retrospect, it made sense that I didn't know how to deal with Joshua's anger. It was his second summer and he was at the height of his tantrums. I was unaware of my angry feelings toward him. In the course of psychiatric treatment and exploration of my feelings, I began to identify first annoyance and later anger as feelings of my own. My headaches began to disappear, and I began liking myself better. Those things didn't happen all at once, or neatly in that order, but today when I get a headache it's usually not severe, and if I think about what's going on around me I can usually identify some angry feelings.

When I first began to express anger to Joshua, guilt would rush right in. After all, how can you get angry with a child, the innocent victim of learning and developmental problems? When I could accept that feelings aren't good or bad, but rather natural emotions, it was easier to be angry with Joshua. My relationship with Joshua may seem stormier now. When I was not aware of my own anger, I had a less honest relationship with him. He would fall accidently when we were together, or by mistake I might bump into him. I always remained calm and I never raised my voice. I kept my real feelings inside. Now I can verbalize and let Joshua know when his obnoxious behavior is not acceptable to me. He yells, "Leave me alone, you're not nice;" or in his best five-year-old terms screams, "You're just a pee-pee, pooh-pooh." I am pleased and proud that he can express his angry feelings.

I still have trouble with anger and often do not deal with it directly. I get it out through physical activity and writing. Over the past five years I've alternated between bicycling, swimming laps, tennis, golf, running and working out in a gym. I like to take some form of physical exercise every day. In the summer I come closest to reaching this. When I first began playing golf, I didn't have the power to hit a ball very far. My instructor said, "Put the face of someone you hate on that ball." My game improved immediately.

Sometimes I still get mixed up with what I feel. I'll watch Joshua playing with other children, who are running around the backyard, throwing and chasing after a ball. Joshua can't keep up, so he goes off by himself or comes back into the house. My throat gets tight and I fight back the tears. Is it hurt or is it anger?

I love you, Joshua,
More and more
    each day
        each week
            each month
                each year.
It's easy for me now,
        to love you
it wasn't always easy.

RELATIONSHIP OF MOTHER AND CHILD

I have always allowed myself the luxury of playing in my mind. Some call it daydreaming or fantasizing or pretending—whatever it's called, I do it. I can still remember the feeling of pregnancy. I liked being pregnant, and feeling my stomach grow. I liked rubbing my stomach and talking to my baby, sharing my dreams for my baby and me. They were dreams of walking barefoot after a spring rain, chasing our shadows on a sunny summer day, catching snowflakes on your tongue, making snow angels in the winter, and crunching through piles of autumn leaves. We'd share some of the fun things I did when I was growing up and some of the things that I'd missed and we'd make up new things to do together. "I sat in the rocking chair in your room today, and I thought, we will share many contented hours, me loving to rock, you loving to be rocked" (excerpt from a diary).

And that never happened. There was a wide gap between my fantasy and reality. Having a baby wasn't instant love for me. To start, it was the primitive relationship of feeding, bathing, and changing diapers. Nursing was pleasurable for me, but my overall feeling for Joshua was one more of responsibility than love. I kept looking for baby magic, the joy of discovery of a hand or some toes, but that didn't happen. Today Joshua is usually a happy child; he has an infectious smile and laughs a lot, but that didn't begin until sometime between year two and year three.

One of the most difficult things for me to learn was judging behavior. Joshua cried a lot and was frustrated easily. How do you distinguish between normal frustration that all children encounter and frustration related to his lack of development?

How do you decide when to intercede and help because he can't help himself, and when not to because he needs to be encouraged to try for himself? I learned by trial and error. Although I often looked to other professionals for answers, *I slowly learned that David and I know our child best.*

If I were with a group of mothers and we put our children together, you might not be aware of Joshua's disability. His differences were subtle. He has learned to do most of the things other children his age can do. The difference is that most children learn to walk, raise their legs, to push or to pull on their own, by trial and error, and Joshua learned because he was taught and encouraged. He is a child who has worked hard every day to accomplish tasks that come naturally for other children.

For the first three years Joshua spent most of his time with me. I nursed him for eight months, then I began to introduce babysitters into his life. There were two important things that got me through that difficult period—a good friend and my car. As Joshua developed, he cried a lot. I tried everything—nursing, changing diapers, singing, rocking, and walking with him. The crying would trigger my own feelings of inadequacy. The car rides relieved Joshua's crying, my friend relieved my self-doubts. He was a good listener. He believed that my feelings were normal and that I was a good mother. I needed that. I needed someone to believe in me as a person at a time when I doubted myself. It was like borrowing a winter coat until the springtime or until you could save to buy one of your own.

As I learned about Joshua, I learned about myself. I learned about meeting my own needs so I could have more to give to him. The more I went out, the more efficient I became at home and the more feelings of love and caring began to take the place of feeling responsible.

In order to keep in touch with Joshua's struggle to learn new tasks, I made it a point to learn something new every year. The first was golf. I had never been athletically inclined, and considered myself uncoordinated. There were two potential benefits in learning golf. First, to get in touch with the complexities of learning a new task, and second, I remember joking about it as a save-the-marriage scheme. David and I were spending little time together. He was working long hours and it seemed as if we had no common interest any more. Golf brought us together for a few hours every week. Golf made me aware of my physical awkwardness.

There was so much to think about; your feet, arms, the club and ball. It was discouraging to try again and again—so many times before experiencing even the smallest success from my efforts. I experienced anxiety in wanting to do well when I played with David. The anxiety, the discouragement, the complexity of all the parts in execution of a single shot which I experienced on the golf course gave me some understanding of Joshua's experiences every hour of every day.

The next year I learned to ride a bicycle. The results were much quicker. This past summer I began jogging. I got discouraged with setbacks, like pains in my legs and inclement weather. It helped me to understand Joshua's struggle.

In arithmetic they teach that the whole is the sum of the parts. For Joshua I look for the parts that make up the while. I break down cooking, cleaning, and laundry into learning tasks for him. Everything we do becomes an informal language lesson too.

One of the fondest memories I have with Joshua is making bread. We might work for weeks or months on a particular skill before we saw changes in Joshua. I had to think of ways to keep my interest up, as well as his. Making bread stands out as one of our best activities. Kneading bread can be hard work. The yeast substance added resistance, and pressing, punching, and pulling the dough were good motor activity for the development of his fingers and hand muscles. We had the immediate reward of yummy odors and fresh baked bread. Joshua enjoyed it. We baked often and had more bread than we needed. Our friends and neighbors were the recipients of the surplus. Later Joshua learned to roll with the rolling pin, decorate with raisins, and choose his own recipients of his originally shaped breads. We never found a person who didn't like our bread. That's a good feeling we both shared.

As Joshua was growing, I was too. I became more confident in my role as a mother. It became easier for me to set limits with him. I was less afraid of making a mistake. I was no longer intimidated by Joshua's tantrums. I could walk away from them, and although they didn't stop, I stopped blaming myself for them. Joshua put me in touch with both aggressive and creative parts of my personality—I felt I could do almost anything if it would help him. I talked the grocery store into selling me wooden coke cartons against their policy and I could return unwanted gifts to the store. (I used to feel intimidated by sales people.) Wooden coke cartons were converted into stairs, tables, chairs, trains, and wagons that required pushing and pulling.

One of the biggest adjustments I had to make was taking the time to let Joshua struggle. It's so much easier to do some task yourself. It would take fifteen seconds to carry him from one room to another—it would take him five minutes to crawl by himself, and I needed to stay in his line of vision so he wouldn't give up and just sit there crying. The minutes quickly added up to hours spent crawling in and out of the back seat of the car and putting on boots. That patience and waiting has never been easy for me.

I also needed to be reminded that just because Joshua had executed a skill did not mean that it was his forever. It was easy for me to forget that once I started hitting the ball over the net, there were still many days when it stopped short. I also have trouble with unrealistic expectations of transference of a skill. Joshua had been fastening snaps for a long time when he got a new pair of trousers. I would get annoyed when he'd come to me saying, "Do this." In reality, these snaps were harder. David and professionals have been helpful to me in overcoming some of my blind spots.

The fulfillment of my prenatal fantasies of making snow angels with Joshua was delayed. Winter brought distress instead of joy. The snow was one more obstacle to overcome. Leg lifting was difficult for Joshua under the best conditions. Adding snow, leggings, and boots made Joshua's first winter walking (his third winter) a tearful one. It was as if he knew his tears would melt the snow around hime for easier walking.

The hurt, frustrations, and disappointments during Joshua's early years were my feelings. These were not his. He was not aware that he was different. It took me some time to work through my feelings and to stop feeling sorry for myself. When I did, loving Joshua was easy. Sometimes I wonder if Joshua has some fantasies on what a mother should be like.

Relationship of Father and Child

He's got a finger next to his thumb that's
five feet long and two feet wide.

When it yells at me, "I mean do it right now!"
I shiver inside.

But attached to his finger is a hand and an
arm that leads to his heart in his middle.
His heart makes me feel warm and happy and giggle.

That's my Daddy.
My Daddy loves me.

Joshua loves his dad and his dad loves Joshua. David is a concerned father. Even when Joshua was a baby and they shared only small amounts of time together, there was never an aspect of Joshua's care that David was unwilling to undertake. He was willing to feed, clothe, or diaper. This past year they have spent a lot of time together. On Saturdays they visit the bakery and health food stores, among other errands. Sometimes Joshua goes to the office with David and always they go out for lunch together. David lets Joshua be a part of what he's doing. If he's washing the car, Joshua has his own sponge; if he's painting a room, Joshua gets a brush and some wall space. From this relationship Joshua gets a feeling of importance. David is also quick to include Joshua's friends on outings.

David has a philosophy of trusting Joshua, expecting that he will behave appropriately. I respect his philosophy and have learned from it. Joshua is eager to please his dad.

Although David has never verbalized it, I think that he had some early fantasies that we never realized, about being a parent and the kinds of things dads do with their children. The three of us vacationed in Florida. It was Joshua's third winter. He cried whenever the sand touched his skin and he was afraid of the waves. The trip was disappointing. Joshua didn't like the sand or the water, and we didn't like all of Joshua's tears.

As Joshua is getting older, I observe him and his dad sharing warm feelings as they do things together. I also observe some ambivalent feelings in David, and occasionally I also observe anxiety. When David is alone with Joshua and it is time for Joshua's medication, David always forgets to give it to him. Or the reason might be, "Well, we were on vacation." Last year David visited Joshua's school. He was not relaxed.

David was sitting with Joshua, trying to get him to complete a task at hand; Joshua's attention was directed at other children in the room. David was unable to engage Joshua's cooperation, and as he kept on trying the teacher observed David's tension and commented that it was affecting Joshua's behavior. When children visit to spend the night, David quizzes them to see what they know and what they can do. A bedtime story becomes a drill session and David seems to be searching for how Joshua compares to others.

One thing is for sure. There isn't anything David wouldn't be willing to do for Joshua.

RELATIONSHIP OF MOTHER AND FATHER

David and I had been married four years prior to Joshua's birth, and although we were not aware of any particular problems in our marriage until after Joshua was born, it was clear to me that our problems were not caused by Joshua.

David is very logical and I am very emotional. We don't understand a lot of things in the same way. After Joshua's first evaluation I remember asking David,

> "How do you feel?"
>
> "Well, I think they have a lot of good suggestions."
>
> "Yes but how do you feel about Joshua's problem?"
>
> "Well, we'll have to try some of those things."
>
> "But how do you feel?"
>
> "I feel like we will do what they suggested."

A major problem in our relationship is communication. As I mentioned earlier, anger has always been a difficult emotion for me to communicate. It is interesting that I married a man who would not permit me to express my anger, or at least highly discouraged me. Now I am aware that this creates emotional dishonesty, and on a tangible level it creates tension.

We've had bad times, we've talked of divorce, and there have been times when we stayed together because neither of us was willing to give up Joshua. There are still a lot of uncertainties between David and me, but there is one thing for sure — whether we stay together as a family or not, Joshua will always have a mother and a father who love him very much.

RELATIVES

One Spring morning Joshua, age two and one-half, David and I reported to the medical genetics department of our state's children's hospital. The morning included chromosome studies and a neurological examination involving four doctors, each a specialist in his own area—genetics, neurology, and child development. During the conference with one of the doctors, I remember being surprised when he addressed himself to our Jewishness. It was his opinion that culturally, Jewish people put education high on their list of values, and that each generation wants their children to have more than they had. He went on to say that Jews do well with extreme problems. They know how to accept and take care of the physically handicapped child, or the severely retarded child, but when it comes to the moderate, nonvisible problems there is difficulty accepting the problem and the child together. The doctor was hypothesizing from his experience. I wasn't able to personalize his comments at the time, but today, two and half years later, I would add two more families to his sampling—David's and mine.

Since our marriage David and I have always lived away from our parents. It forced us to face our problems with Joshua together, making decisions on medical help without emotional involvement of family.

On a conscious level I believe both of our families would say they accept the fact that Joshua has a problem, but I think their behavior contradicts that, and at best their feelings are ambivalent. I remember a telephone conversation with my mother. It was a couple of months after Joshua's initial evaluation. I had been working with him for almost eight weeks, not long enough to see any tangible results. I was feeling scared and uncertain about him and about me. One evening I was talking with my mother and she asked if we had received the written report from Joshua's evaluation. As I began reporting some information, I got choked up and started to cry. After I composed myself I said, "Mom, what I need from you now is just to know that you love me." She responded, "Do you think I wouldn't love you because of Joshua?" Her response had nothing to do with my request. I think that was what the doctor had meant about not being able to accept the child and the problem together.

Another pattern that began to appear with our families was a way they had of discounting Joshua's problem. I think they would call it "trying to reassure us that everything's OK." It went something like this:

Question to family member: "What do you think is wrong with Joshua? He can't run."

Family response: "Do you want him to be a football player? Besides, your nephew's not coordinated either."

Question: "What else? His speech is not developing."

Family response: "I've already told you about Einstein."

My mother-in-law would call and say, "Hello, how's Joshua, everything's fine isn't it?" I don't think it mattered whether I said yes or no, because her response was usually the same: "Yes, well, I'm glad, and I think everything's going to be all right." On one visit my mother-in-law asked if there was any of "that" on my side of the family. My mother had already made it clear that in all probability it was the poor medical care Joshua received at birth. Another time my mother-in-law confided to me that she never told her brother about Joshua, and assured me she wasn't saying much to her family. She evaluated people on their educational background, how far they've gone in school and what schools they've attended. It must be difficult for her to accept a child with a questionable educational future. It is tempting to conclude that Joshua is a disappointment to her grandmotherly fantasies.

I think that both of our families have done the best that they could in a difficult situation. When my parents see Joshua they are attracted to his warm and loving personality, and I think my mother-in-law would help in any way she could. This year she paid the majority of Joshua's school tuition.

A SPECIAL RELATIONSHIP

I'm writing this in the basement of my home and upstairs I hear bursts of laughter and running and more laughter. That's Joshua and Betty. Betty is our babysitter, confidante, and friend. She is truly a gift from God. Our family met Betty more than five years ago and she babysat for us occasionally. When Joshua was beginning his second year of school I was working parttime and needed some dependable child care arrangements. It was our good fortune that Betty was available. She loves all children and Joshua soon became a special part of her heart. She loves him free of charge. There isn't anything he has to do to make it with her. She offers him patience; she will read the same story a hundred times if Joshua asks and plays games that are worn with use, always with fresh enthusiasm. She has patience and flexibility.

Betty loves me and I love her. She accepts me. I can be sad and cry with her and not have to tell her why I am sad. I accept Betty. She can talk of a painful moment in her past and cry. I can hug her and hold her. Best of all we laugh together and share childlike secrets. Betty sees David and me as devoted parents to a wonderful child. I like to remember those words when I don't feel devoted and Joshua's not acting so wonderful.

Betty has given Joshua another loving friend, Carl, a man who is slightly less than fifty years of age and is disabled from a hip injury. Carl drives for Betty and picks Joshua up from school two afternoons a week. Carl has grown to love Joshua too. You can see it in the cards he sends on Halloween and special gifts he wraps for him for no special occasion at all. In the summertime Carl drives over to the house to play ball with

Joshua, and if Joshua wants to eat at Betty's house, Carl's right there for pickup and delivery. They have their own private jokes, and Carl calls Joshua on the telephone and Joshua calls him back.

Betty and Carl see Joshua as nothing less than perfect. They describe him as bright, witty, and taking his time in being a child. They do see his difficulty with running and hand coordination and work with him. I think their love and acceptance and belief in Joshua have been important factors in contributing to Joshua's self-esteem and progress.

ONLY CHILD: RELATIONSHIP WITH SELF

David wanted a large family and the professionals were recommending having another child. I was in conflict. There's a part of me that gets excited about creating a new life and remembering the warm feelings of nursing a baby. Yet there was another part of me that said no! You don't have a baby if the marriage isn't good. I didn't know of any babies that saved relationships. So Joshua remained an only child.

For his first four years Joshua showed no awareness of himself as being different from anyone else. His personality changed during that time. As a baby he cried a lot and was content to sit looking blankly into space. He became an attractive child who had a winning way with adults. His smiles warmed the cold and the grumpy. He was liked everywhere he went.

The year before Joshua started school we worked daily on his physical, motor, language, and sensory development. He was not a self-starter. He required prodding and encouragement. For even the slightest move toward self-help, Joshua was rewarded. He also got a lot of loving "just because." This love worked for and against him. He was feeling very good about himself, and that's good. He walked into school shortly before his third birthday with the attitude "you know you love me and there isn't anything I have to do to make it with you but smile and flirt a little with my eyes." That was the bad part. Interaction meant work and effort on Joshua's part. If he was around adults and other children, unless I interceded he could persuade someone to hold him on his or her lap so he could be the inactive observer. We had to work at participation.

Between the ages of four and five, Joshua became aware of himself in relation to other children. A question like, "Mommy, why can't I run like Jimmy?" or a defiant, "I won't do it" (cut with scissors) were clues that he was becoming more aware of himself.

Joshua has a shy part to his personality that often surprises the people around him. Anxiety causes him to withdraw with his two favorite fingers in his mouth.

By the age of five adults had lost their number one spot, and Joshua's peers became more important to him. At school his teacher had reported that the other children liked him but he was shy and not aware of his own acceptance into the group. Perhaps this is one of the liabilities of being an only child. Being sensitive to this problem, I have made an effort to find other children for Joshua to play with. Before I started working I would take him to a babysitter who had other children to care for, rather than bring a babysitter to our home. One summer I joined the co-op group with four other mothers. One day a week I was responsible for the planning and care of six other children in our home. It was good for Joshua to learn to share his things. Three days a week he played at the other children's homes, and we had one day together.

Being an only child has had some financial advantages — not taking away from other children's needs. But our expenses are higher than those of parents with an average child. Neurological examinations are $50, EEG tests $35, blood tests $60, psychological tests run from $30 to $200, and school tuition is $150 a month. These have become fixed and expected expenses.

LEARNING DISABILITY

I had just picked Joshua up from school, and we were passing our dentist's office when he pointed out, "That's my teeth doctor." He paused and added, "I have lots of doctors, don't I, Mommy?" He began to list the dentist, his pediatrician, the neurologist, and a psychologist who had recently tested him. He's also been seen by a child development specialist, a genetics specialist, a speech and hearing therapist, and an educational therapist. Joshua's right — he has seen many doctors, Ph.D.s and M.D.s. all describing him using different terms — learning disability, mental retardation, minimal brain dysfunction, hypotonic, hyperactive, developmental delay and cerebral palsy.

A written report followed Joshua's first evaluation:

"Joshua is a handsome and social boy, 29 months, who was referred by his parents because of slow motor development. The family has been aware of this for more than a year. From testing and observations, he is currently performing considerably below age level. He is essentially non-verbal and depends upon gestures for comprehension. Curiosity is minimal and the information he receives from his feedback systems appears to be low. Awareness of himself and what he can do is questionable. He is dependent on his parents and exercises no individuality or personality of his own, except for the word "Mine."

The biggest question at this time was what would happen to the gap between Joshua's actual performance and the expected performance for children his age. Would it get bigger, stay the same or decrease? The same label meant different things to me at different times—it depended on my emotional state as well as my understanding. It also depended on the frame of reference of the person using it. We are dropping the labels. They are more confusing than helpful, as their meaning varies from person to person, whether professional or layman. Labels can hurt. If you tell a child that he's retarded, he will probably be compliant and act dumb. I think one reason why Joshua continues to learn and grow is because it is expected of him.

The balancing act is in continuing our expectations without putting too much pressure on him. Last week I was talking with the director of Joshua's school. She told me that a doctor who is a school consultant asked her to prepare David and me to accept having a retarded child. She agreed. That was a year and a half ago. Today she believes that that evaluation is no longer valid. With that kind of history and progress, it would be dangerous to predict Joshua's future.

Joshua was five years, two months old when we received the last report:

"You have a child who is not grossly impaired....He has obviously positive social attributes...He does have some things that are not entirely normal for his age...His greatest deficit is motor execution. We have eliminated emotional causes and environmental deprivation as causes for the deficit....There are a number of subtleties that make one suspicious of organic neurological abnormalities."

At age five, for the first time, we heard the term "average." It referred to two subtests on the last psychological testing. One was in the area of language. I picked up on that word immediately and we were warned by the test interpreter not to generalize. The important point was that Joshua had come a long way.

As parents it is often difficult to find out what is wrong and right with your child. David and I have attended all of the testing evaluations. Some were helpful, others were not. Sometimes I get the feeling that professionals think we're retarded. The last time I was asked to sign a release of information statement, I asked if I could put my name on the list of persons the report would be sent to. The response was, "No, the way it gets written up you, as parents, probably wouldn't understand it anyway." My response was, "Well, teach me then, I want to understand." My unspoken feeling was anger for being discounted.

We have received some written reports. When they come

children diving into the water, running, racing and climbing. I want my child to be free to race and play with other children. I wonder if the Pepsi company knows some mothers cry when their commercial comes on. I do.

Diary Entry: November 1975

Today was your birthday, Joshua; you were five years old. I think I will always remember this morning. How you ran into the bedroom, naked, with your arms outstretched, saying, "Look at me Mommy, I'm five and I'm not big." I've photographed your look of disappointment, your frustrated "What do we do now," like acid dropped onto a zinc plate.

As I sit here writing in my diary, I think how much we are alike. Your birthday is a milestone. You expect things to be different on those days. Like the day you were born, after carrying you inside of me for nine months. I thought on the day you were born I would love you. You were exciting and interesting and scary to me...but I was disappointed. I didn't feel the love I expected. You are now a lovable child, Joshua, and I love you. I don't know when it happened I didn't notice it on any particular day. I think it's like your being big.

As I am writing in my diary, I'm writing to you because it's your day and the fifth anniversary of our day of departure from each other and the beginning for you to become you.

Where are you now, Joshua? You have come a long way. You do so many things by yourself. You go off to school every day and tell me on your way out the door, "I'm going to have a good day today, Mommy." You smile a lot now.

The most exciting thing for me is thinking that three years ago, no one would have predicted that you would be talking nonstop, telling "knock, knock" jokes, and singing "Rudolph, The Red Nose Reindeer" in July. They even have different labels for you now. I don't mind labels if they're used in helping us to learn to work with you and if you can wear them like clothes and discard them when they no longer serve the purpose. Just as I don't know what fashion will be in style five years from now, I don't know what labels will be used to describe you or how you will be the same or how you will be different five years from today.

We have our good times together, like swimming in the summer and baking on Friday afternoons in the winter. We have our bad times too, when no matter what happens you say, "That won't do" and get frustrated and angry and cry and kick and hit. Sometimes I get frustrated and angry and tell you to "Go upstairs, get away from me, we can't make it together right now."

I've learned that I can't meet all of your needs, Joshua, and so I find people who can. How lucky we are to have Betty who is like an extended family member, and our good friend Carl.

Sometimes I wonder what effect all the times I leave you has. I do that a lot now. I meditate and I like that you've learned to be quiet during that time. I take a yoga class and I jog in the morning and sometimes I'll get a babysitter for you so I can take off for an afternoon alone on my bicycle. Sometimes I even go away by myself for a weekend. I need my alone time, Joshua, time away from you, away from Dad, away from work and school. I need time to rest, to think, to get some distance and perspective. Sometimes I use the time to stop thinking and just rest or have fun.

I see you're starting to do some things on your own, too. You like sleeping overnight at Jim's and eating supper at Betty's and Carl's. And how well you liked traveling across the state with Betty to spend Christmas with her family, and how you are talking about your next trip by yourself: "Just me and Betty." You really know how to have fun and laugh and be silly. I like playing balloon with you and laughing and being silly.

This has been a long entry, and a very special day, with your birthday, picnic, ice cream and cake and presents and wishes. My wish for you, on this day, is that you can hold on to your happiness. My wish for your dad and me is that we can let you grow and be what you want to be and not what we want to make you. Today showed promise of a good year and the hope of a good life.

"Goodnight, Joshua, Mommy loves you."

TIM

Tim's mother and father wanted to contribute varying points of view about their experiences with their hyperactive son, both to exemplify the conflicts from different vantage points and to show the cooperation and essential strategies that gradually developed between them as parents. Beginning as a colicky child who drove his parents to daily distraction, Tim has blossomed now in intellectual ability. While still having some problems with writing skills, his main deficiencies are attention span, poor coordination, and social control. A most important difficulty these parents of a first baby faced was simply their lack of knowledge of what to expect from a child, normal or otherwise. Tim has a three-year-old brother.

The thought of writing about our problems with Tim is perplexing. If we dwell on all the negative things we feel, you will think we don't love him. What are our true feelings? We bounce back and forth between love and hate, compassion and bitterness, optimism and disappointment, hope and resentment. We are not at peace about how to handle a hyperactive child! How do we dare act like we are experts? Thus, this opening paragraph becomes somewhat of a disclaimer to the effect that you, the reader, should interpret this as one view from two struggling parents who make no claims to having the answers.

MOTHER

It is often said that some couples go into marriage with visions of total bliss and joy, with never a thought of strains and difficulties. We went into parenthood with the same false impressions.

I remember after three years of marriage we decided we'd like to have a baby. After a year of trying, we consulted an obstetrician. He had me check my temperature every morning to determine ovulation. This didn't work, so he did some tests to see if everything was OK physically.

Finally after some more advice and another year I became pregnant. The day we found out, we celebrated by going out for lunch. We couldn't have been more elated.

Everything about the pregnancy seemed normal. There were a lot of backaches and some swelling in my legs during the last three months, but it all seemed a normal part of being pregnant.

At six o'clock one summer morning I was awakened by a gush of water. We knew this was the time. I was scared. We called the doctor's office at nine and he told me to come right in.

The doctor examined me and told me that my water had broken and within a few hours I would start having labor pains. Well, I waited all day, but no pains. We went to bed about eleven that night. By that time my back was aching so much I couldn't lie down. At 1:00 a.m. we called the doctor again. He told me to go to the hospital. By 3:10 that afternoon, after thirty three hours of dry labor, our son was born. Tim was the product of an eight and one-half month pregnancy. His birth weight was eight pounds, three ounces, and he was twenty two inches long.

FATHER

His delivery was very difficult because he was face down and forceps were required. We went to classes so the husband could be in the delivery room. We practiced the breathing techniques. What a waste of time! With the baby face down the pain was constant. I shall never forget the look of total exhaustion on my wife after that delivery as they brought her back from the delivery room. Then I started to understand the sacrifices a parent makes for a child.

MOTHER

We watched as the nurses held him and noticed that he didn't cry. We remember worrying about whether he was alive. There was difficulty in getting Tim to start breathing.

Because of the difficulty I had in giving birth, I did not want or couldn't even hold Tim when they brought him in to be fed. Most of the time the nurses fed him: I couldn't sit up.

Towards the end of the week I was able to feed Tim some of the time. When the nurses would bring him in, they would often comment that he was the "best baby in the nursery."

At the end of seven days I dressed Tim for coming home. He was screaming all the time. By the time we were in the car and on our way home both of us were crying. I know now I should have stayed in the hospital another day or so. I was still very weak and tired. The crying was only the beginning.

The next months were like a nightmare. Tim would fuss most of the day except when he napped. During the night feedings, we would pray that he could go back to sleep. Tim was so colicky that he would cry and fuss two hours before we could get him back to sleep. Then he would be awake in two hours for another feeding.

Both of us were exhausted. It seemed we were always giving Tim a bottle. It took half an hour to feed and burp him and then a couple of hours to get him back to sleep. During this time we were each getting about six hours sleep a night. It did not take long before exhaustion started setting in.

Sometimes he would fall asleep taking his bottle. We would carefully put him into his crib and he would immediately awaken screaming and spitting up. Even during the day he would be very irritable when he was awake. We became frantic. We were always very tired.

I started resenting what Tim was doing to me and to our

lives. I felt he was giving me no peace, no time for myself or for us. It seemed each of us had the answers for the other. We had never had so many problems and disagreements before Tim.

I would call Tim's pediatrician three or four times a week during the first weeks of Tim's life. Always, I was hoping for a magic cure for his extreme fussiness.

Some of the suggestions we tried were valium for calmness, colic drops, and lactic acid to break down the fats in the formula. The colic drops did help some, but Tim remained a fussy baby. Our only other hope was that, according to the baby books, colic passes after three months.

Being a mother for the first time, I know I was very nervous and overreacted much of the time. But I realize now that it would be impossible for almost anyone to be calm when a baby cries most of the day and night.

BOTH PARENTS

We talked with friends with older children looking for answers and comfort. Most replies would be that he'll be much better after three months.

Colic continued for nine months. Tim was sleeping through the two o'clock feeding by three months, but he was up at six o'clock and still fussing during his waking hours. It seemed we could do nothing to please or comfort him.

Tim was not very alert to his surroundings. He seemed listless and unaware of his mobile or toys. But at the time we didn't realize this was unusual, especially since he was our first child.

We have some friends who have a boy four months older than Tim. Each time we were with them we could see such an expanding difference in their general progress.

The fussiness and irritability continued on after the first year. When Tim learned to sit alone, I remember always having to locate him on a huge blanket because of his projectile vomiting. Nevertheless he was a good eater. He couldn't wait for the food to be put into his mouth.

Tim was slow to learn large motor skills such as crawling, pulling himself up on a chair, or sitting up. He seemed like a listless blob. His eyes did not seem to focus on anything. We notice this most with the mobile on his bed—it was as if it were not there. He just did not seem to be aware of what was going on around him. The doctor told us to put him on his stomach on the floor so he could practice pushing up. He would scream all the time he was in that position and never pushed himself up, at least until much later on.

During his second year Tim had extreme diarrhea. It was day in and day out—perhaps five or six times a day. The father reacted most to this. It seemed like the focal point of his life was changing runny, stinking diapers. The doctor recommended putting him on a milk- and gluten (wheat and flour) -free diet.

We were so frustrated with the colic and diarrhea problems that at one point, on the doctor's advice, we decided to have him checked completely at the hospital for a few days. We packed Tim up and put him in the car. We started out and while driving we kept looking at him sitting in the back seat so peacefully and quietly. How could we leave that baby in the hospital alone? It was tearing our hearts out. What a dilemma! We were so desperate for help while we had him at home, but could not bear the thought of leaving him at the hospital. We turned around and went home! After about a year the problem of the extreme diarrhea cleared up.

The worst problem of all was (and is) the irritability. This child never seems to be satisfied. The mother's main thought was that as a mother she was a complete failure. She couldn't do anything to help the child or make him happy. It seemed that his main goal in life was to hang around his mother and fuss and whine. The main thought of the father at this time was that if the mother would be more strict with the child, the problems would go away. He always seemed more content and better behaved with his father. We have found out since that most children react this way at that age—fussy and whiny with mother, but calm with father. As time went on he stabilized (that word may not be appropriate) in the sense that he was fussy and whiny with both parents.

The strain between us as parents was great. Each would blame the other for lack of discipline. We were frantic to be away to renew our relationship, and we were very lucky to have that opportunity. It was like we each lived two personalities. One with and one without Tim. Those times away were precious, if for nothing else than to be reassured of our love for one another. We didn't take Tim with us much because any change seemed to make him more irritable. Plus, we could never be relaxed when we took him. No one seemed to believe us, especially relatives. The responses were usually "There is nothing wrong with him," or "He'll outgrow it." We began thinking we were losing our minds, and felt even more inadequate.

After Tim's second year we felt there definitely was something wrong with this child. It was evident comparing him to other children his own age. He was beginning to have tantrums. They would last for five minutes or so, and would occur seven or eight times a day. The tantrums were provoked for what seemed to us unimportant reasons. The TV would have a mechanical disorder and he would through a fit. It was time to wash his hands and he would throw a fit. Out of the blue he would decide he wanted to watch "Sesame Street." If it did not happen to be on just at that moment, he would throw a fit. It seemed as if he could be happy one minute and then go into a screaming rage the next minute.

By the time Tim was three we had enrolled him in a cooperative nursery school. This we thought would be the answer to Tim's problem. Maybe he needed children his own age to play with more than just at church on Sundays. Much to our dismay things got worse. Tim just couldn't seem to handle the large group of children. It was even worse the days I participated. He would pull toys away from kids and upset boxes of pegs and other toys. He was continually in a crying rage.

MOTHER

I, as a mother, dreaded the days I helped because of these

things. I would often have to leave the room because I was crying. Whenever I would go to another room of the nursery school Tim would come crying. I could not get away from him!

One of the nursery school teachers thought Tim had an extreme mother complex because he was always wanting to be with me. Being with me wouldn't have been too bad, but he was never happy. He always fussed about something. We made a great effort to have Tim do many things with his dad so he would relate to him. This was not the answer either. He was still the same—always wanting to fuss and whine at his mother. Only in later years (six and older) did he start relating more to his father.

BOTH PARENTS

By the end of the nursery school year we felt even more convinced that Tim needed some special help. We were sure we just couldn't possibly have made such huge mistakes in raising what seemed to be a "bratty" child. Tim acted like some of the spoiled children we all have heard and read about.

We met with Tim's nursery school teacher for an end-of-the-year conference. She told us of a psychologist who dealt with children who had special needs. This was when we learned of learning disabilities.

In the meantime our second baby was born. Delivery was much easier with this child. But needless to say, we wondered whether we could be able to cope with another baby.

Tim was tested by the psychologist at age three years and nine months. Although he was found to be functioning within the normal range of intelligence, difficulties were found in the areas of language comprehension and expression, short-term memory, attention span, and fine and gross motor coordination. Although Tim was very friendly and cooperative, all of his actions were impulsive and he chattered constantly. After about one-half hour of tests, hyperventilation (heavy breathing), distractibility, and physical activity markedly increased. It was also concluded that there might be mild motor impairment in addition to hyperactivity.

The recommendations were:

1. A medication trial should be considered.
2. In the fall, Tim would benefit from enrollment at a special preschool with small classes and the availability of strong language development program.
3. Close supervision and consistency in managing his behavior were a necessity. We were to isolate him for intolerable negative behaviors such as temper tantrums, and we were to endeavor to overlook minor negative behaviors.
4. With respect to nighttime toilet accidents, parents were advised to keep Tim in training pants rather than diapers at night, to decrease liquids in late afternoon and evening, to provide the bulkiest meal in morning and noon.
5. A follow-up evaluation was planned in four to six weeks to check effectiveness of medication.

When we received the results of this evaluation, the mother was relieved to know that she wasn't the cause of the behavior problems we were having with Tim. She felt compassion for this child, and felt this would be the beginning of our helping him.

The father reacted quite differently, though. His ego had been hurt. He couldn't seem to realize the fact that something was really wrong with his son. Most of this reaction was because I, as the father, blamed my wife for most of the child's problems, thinking that she was not strict enough with the child. My ego was hurt because my diagnosis had been completely in error and because of the shock of having a child with a problem. My reaction was "That will never happen to me." I pitied myself for awhile and was sort of angry at life for dealing me this blow. I finally decided to pick myself up, grab on to the problem, and fight it. The feelings of anger and pity passed soon. Many fathers, we have found, can never seem to admit there is a difficulty. So the mother has the problem to deal with, without her husband's support. Believe us, *both* parents have to work together in order to help this type of child and in order to survive themselves!

Hyperactivity takes many different forms. In Tim's case he was extremely irritable as a baby. As he became older he would be very happy one minute, and the next he would be crying and screaming for no apparent reason. Short attention span was also evident; he just did not stick with an activity for very long.

It seems that no matter what we mention for him to do, he'll be very unhappy and reply that he wants to do the opposite. If we have eggs for breakfast, he whines and replies, "Well, I wish I could have cereal," or vice versa.

Our son is very fidgety. He "flips" his hands and rolls on the floor. He also will knock his silverware on the floor or sit and kick the table or chair leg while he is eating. Another sign we notice with Tim is his incessant talking. He cannot seem to quit talking. He always is demanding an answer or reply.

In some ways Tim seemed to be advanced. He learned his *ABC's* quite early, and he also had a great interest in numbers and counting. These things occurred when he was about two and one-half years old.

We remember hearing people talk of the different stages a child goes through such as "terrible two's," "trusting three's," "fascinating four's," "and fabulous five's." When Tim was two, he acted the same as he did when he was one and the same when he was three, four, and five. We were always in the "terrible two's"! We were always waiting for things to improve with age.

The psychologist who tested Tim was also the psychologist for a special nursery school and kindergarten for children who have learning disabilities and who are hyperactive. She and the director of the school believed that Tim would benefit from the special school.

In July 1974 Tim went to a morning program at the school. During this summer period the school was a day camp rather than an academic program. Then in the fall we enrolled him in this special school for the morning nursery program. The class was small, maybe eight children and a teacher and an adult helper, plus volunteers. Tim attended five mornings a week.

Tim really didn't mind going, but the time there was difficult for him. Even though Tim was four, his emotional age was about two. He spent most of his mornings crying because things weren't going his way. The teacher would help him work through these periods of being out of control.

The director of the school thought it might be well to have Tim checked by a neurologist. We were seeing Tim roll his eyes back and blinking often. He was also stuttering some and forgetting something he had just said. We would also have frequent outbursts of screaming and crying over frustrations he should have been able to handle at his age.

The main findings from the neurologist were that Tim had an enlarged head and he was having subclinical seizures. These are seizures such as an epileptic would have, but are minor in nature, so there is little outer display of their effects. Tim was started on medication, which stopped the eye rolling and the outbursts for the most part. Tim also started sleeping better at night. Before the medication he would awaken three or four times a night crying and trembling.

At the end of the school year Tim was tested again. The test results at four years and eleven months showed Tim was functioning within normal intellectual range, with nonverbal reasoning significantly higher than linguistic ability. He has difficulty understanding the underlying structure of complex sentences and questions. Tim's visual perception and nonverbal reasoning (such as working mazes) are excellent. He has difficulties in smooth continuous motor coordination—that is, he is clumsy at large motor skills such as running and jumping, and his fine motor skills such as writing are ragged and broken. He continues to have difficulties in delay of gratification (getting something that gives him pleasure) and frustration tolerance (sharing, waiting his turn).

It is important that Tim fully understand instructions and explanations prior to responding. At home, expectations should be clear and consistent, but coupled with praise and encouragement for his efforts. As Tim requires large amounts of individual attention, daily schedules should be planned so he receives attention for appropriate rather than inappropriate behavior. Verbal instructions and explanations should be as brief and concrete as possible and he should be given advance warning of any change in routine.

Again he attended the summer program in July. The children did a lot of outdoor activities. Swimming was always included. The program was mainly to help develop motor skills and to help the child gain social skills.

During the following year we sought further help to try to get the problem under control. We asked the director of Tim's school to recommend a child psychologist. During the first visit he talked to each of us individually, including Tim. He was gathering information about our backgrounds. All seemed to be going well, but then he started wanting us to bring our second child and all of us to spend time together in his office. We were usually worn out by the time we got there and it was nerve-wracking, but we kept hoping we would get some help. What a farce! At $40 an hour, and after spending $240, we arrived one afternoon, got into the office only to have the man say, "Well, what do you want to talk about today?" Damn — $240 and he asks us what we want to talk about, Doesn't he know by now? The crowning blow was the comment he made one day to the effect that he did not believe there were hyperactive children. We never went back!

Having had more time pass, we see that the person who has helped us the most is the school's director and we are eternally grateful to her. She has seen Tim more on a day-in-day-out basis. We believe that the only kind of people who can really help are those who are or have been in the situation with a child who has learning disabilities.

Tim went into a first year kindergarten program. He made a lot of improvement in a year. (Each child in the class works at his own level.) The children were helped to have frequent successes and were praised often. Tim was able to work on something for a short period of time. He still demanded much of our time and wanted to be with his mother as much as possible.

One of the hardest things for us to overcome is the feeling of not accomplishing anything with Tim. He is so very negative and complains so much about everything. We can never seem to do much to please him in simple ways that most children are pleased. For the first half hour before breakfast it is very normal to hear whining concerning four or five small issues about which Tim is unhappy. For instance, Tim comes downstairs and his mother is setting the table. He'll start fussing because he wanted to set the table. If he forgets to brush his teeth, he'll stomp and whine because he had to do it or argue about doing it another time. Or his mother will cook soft eggs and he'll complain because he doesn't have cereal, or vice versa. So go our days.

Many of these things sound like almost any child at one time or another, we know. But in a hyperactive child the problems occur *many, many* times a day. Because of the continuous occurrence each day, it is difficult to be on top.

All parents must try to be consistent, but with a hyperactive child consistency is much more important. Another important strategy is to try to remain calm when talking to the child. The more excited we get the more anxious he gets and the harder it is to bring him under control.

We have found that spankings rarely are beneficial punishment. Isolation from the rest of the family seems to be the best for Tim. We send him to his room for five minutes. When we first started this, Tim was in his room many times in the course of the day. But he seldom has to be sent now.

Many times we are so full of anger and so very tense that Tim senses it and he becomes completely out of control. Then we must calm ourselves first and talk as quietly and calmly as possible to him. Again, parents of "normal" children can say, "That's what all parents must do—isolate the child, be calm and consistent!" It's true, but with hyperactive children it is *doubly* important to do these things.

Because Tim is very negative about himself, he needs much encouragement and praise. If possible, we try to set up success experiences for him. He really wants to please and feels great about himself when a positive experience happens. Most of the time it would seem he is doing everything he can to create problems. We try to realize this is really not his intention.

Another idea that helps Tim is to let him do chores at home. He likes to set the table, unload the dishwasher, empty wastebaskets, and vacuum. One of us has to stay with him while he's doing these things; and he can't be hurried.

MOTHER

I, as the mother, am very blessed to have a husband who has genuine interest in his family and who helps me tremendously. His working schedule is such that he works in his office at home part time. He is usually home during the critical hours before dinner and up until bedtime.

When I clean up the kitchen he has the boys. In the summer they are outside taking walks, playing, or just sitting. In the winter they run errands during that time.

After breakfast my husband reads the paper and supervises the boys while I clean the kitchen, make beds, and spend time to myself reading.

Our evenings are very important to the two of us. It's the only time we can be together to talk or read or watch television. Unlike most families we have no family discussion at the dinner table. It is a very trying and hectic time for all.

Another way for us to cope is by having an afternoon and early evening out. We try to have a sitter on Saturday or Sunday afternoon if possible. It doesn't have to be an expensive time. Just shopping, sitting together and talking uninterrupted, or going on a picnic can help us come back to the situation refreshed.

Putting the children to bed and eating later can be another way to help renew ourselves.

We are fortunate to be able to take several short trips during the year. These trips have done wonders for our relationship. Even if parents could manage one night away at a motel in their town, I'm sure they could return to face the next weeks with a better attitude. I would cut down on the food budget and clothes budget, or any budget, in order to be away once every month or two.

Good sitters are hard to find if grandparents aren't able or live too far away. But keep looking and asking. Sometimes churches know of people or colleges have girls who want extra money. Or even young married couples enjoy this way to earn extra income.

If possible, it is important for the mother to have some work, hobby, or other activity (away from home if possible) to help her cope. The mother needs to have her mind filled with thoughts other than the problem of her child. If she is away part of a day at least once a week, she can hopefully come back refreshed and ready to start again.

FATHER

I was raised in a home where the roles of mother and father were clear cut and quite separate. The mother did all the housework including the care and feeding of the children, together with their educational and moral upbringing. The father was the breadwinner, and apart from duties such as lawn mowing and mechanical repairs, he *never* did anything with the children. While I am not intentionally trying to be a chauvinist, such a family atmosphere had to affect my expectations of being a father. This, coupled with the presence of a hyperactive child, put a tremendous amount of strain upon my wife, until I finally woke up to the special problems we faced and the need for more involvement on my part.

I see my role now as part of a team with my wife, trying to give each other enough breaks and relief so that we can cope with our family situation. Each person has a "patience threshold," and I think my wife and I are reasonably patient people, but the demands of Tim frequently push us beyond this threshold. We often exceed the threshold, but our goal is not to.

On a typical day I usually start off by getting at least one of the children dressed in the morning. My wife finds herself under strain shortly after breakfast. During this time I take the children to the family room for supervised play while she takes some time for herself to do morning chores. When I go to work she attempts to watch the children and try to do household duties. Tim attends nursery school and gets home around 3 p.m. By the time I arrive home and have supper, about 5 p.m., my wife has really felt the strain. With the tiredness I feel, and the children feel, it is not unreasonable for us to categorize the time between 5 p.m. and 7 p.m. (bedtime) as the worst experience of the day. What was the solution? It seems to work well for me, as tired as I might be, to remove the children from being with my wife. In the summer I take them for walks, or fishing, or some other activity. In the winter I try to use that time for errands, such as shopping, car repairs, and so on. This is so much better than trying to supervise the children in a closed room, especially when one of them is hyperactive.

My wife and I are also fortunate enough to take trips together that allow us to renew and reinforce our relationship. This is very important. You must have time alone even if this means staying in a hotel in your hometown or having dinner late after the children are in bed.

To summarize, the father can help greatly by getting involved.

A strong communicative base is also important in coping with this problem. I would like to have a dime for every hour we have spent discussing our problems with Tim. While we often wonder if we can't find something else to talk about, these discussions have been helpful.

To me experiences with a child such as this run hot and cold, but never in between. There are times when you feel the warmth, the closeness. Then there are times when you want to withdraw completely because of the strain. Every morning I get up determined to handle Tim better. But every day carries with it the strain that discharges my determination.

As has been stated, my feelings bounce back and forth. I so often start out doing something with Tim with such a positive attitude, and end up with a bitter nightmare experience. Here is an example of what happens: As mentioned earlier, I often take Tim to the shopping center to relieve my wife. Following is the typical dialogue and my reactions as they are and how I am really feeling on the inside:

Riding in the Car

TIM: What are those buttons and dials for on the dashboard?

DAD: Those are the speedometer and gas gauge and other things.

DAD: (inside) Here we go again; everytime we get in the car the same sequence of questions.

TIM: Dad, you are out of gas, we'd better stop and get some.

DAD: We have plenty of gas. The needle is on F.

DAD: (inside) He wants, of course, to stop at the gas station. He seems to never be happy to do the things we left the house for.

TIM: How many errands are we going to run?

DAD: Just one, Tim.

TIM: But, we always do just one.

DAD: (inside) Always this same sequence of questions. Why can't he be happy to go to the shopping center? We often run more than one errand, but if less I always get the same reaction.

TIM: This car sure is dirty. We had better get it washed.

DAD: We are just going to the shopping center! Do you have it straight?

TIM: (sulking, head in hands) Yes.

DAD: (inside) That kid bugs the hell out of me! Just like a little old lady! Why can't he be happy to go to the shopping center?

TIM: Dad, you are speeding.

DAD: No, Tim you are reading the RPM gauge instead of the speed gauge.

DAD: (inside) He always does this too, but try to bear up as this is the way a child like this is. Be calm!

Arriving at the shopping center.

TIM: How many stores are we going to?

DAD: Three.

TIM: Rats!

DAD: (inside) There would never be a big enough number.

Inside the shopping center.

TIM: (walking by children's clothing) I wished I had toughskins pants.

DAD: Mom just bought you three pairs!

TIM: But I want some blue ones

DAD: (inside) He already has red, green and brown! There is never enough to satisfy that kid.

TIM: (walking by the candy counter) I wished I had some peanuts.

DAD: No, Tim, we are *not* going to buy anything special.

DAD: (inside) Why can't he just walk along and keep his mouth shut, or talk about something that isn't in the form of a request?

TIM: (walking by the toy department after father has completed his purchase) I wished I had a six-million-dollar man.

DAD: Tim, we are not going to buy anything special! Do not ask again! If you do I will take you to the car. Do you hear me? Do you have it straight?

DAD: (inside) I wish I was the six-million-dollar man. I would either fly out of here or be able to give this demanding child the love and patience he needs. What a rotten father I am! I never should have had any kids! I am not fit for them!

TIM: (later at another store, having battled to keep quiet for awhile) I would like to get my picture taken.

DAD: No, Tim

DAD: (inside) I have had it! I had some more shopping to do, but I think I will go home. Maybe it will be bedtime.

Arriving home.

DAD: Tim, it is time for bed. Please go upstairs and get your pajamas on.

TIM: But I want a drink.

DAD: OK, but hurry up!

DAD: (inside) I know! I know! You should not hurry a child like this. My wife will remind me again about this after Tim is in bed. I have just had it!

I am sure, if you are parents, that isolated instances of the above behaviors have occurred with your children, but it is the continuous exposure to them that puts me beyond my patience threshold.

BOTH PARENTS

In the last few months the director of Tim's school has gotten a key across to us for helping Tim—LOVE.— more than we thought we could ever give. We have been having many rewarding and warm experiences with Tim by trying to strip away pestering him for minor negative behaviors and really praising him for positive behaviors. It is amazing how well he has responded. He really does want to please. Another blessing occurred. Last year his IQ testing found him very much average around 100. This year he tested at 121. He is reading and doing math at the second grade, third month level. He is in first grade. We are very thankful.

But the most important information she gave us is that Tim needs lots of love. He needs much more praise than most children. He needs to be praised for things that seem trite to us. She recommended that we "Get off his back!" Ignore the squirming and excessive chatter. These are things he cannot control.

We have been working very hard to find the things that Tim does well and reward or praise him immediately. It becomes easier all the time (part of this is his getting older). He just glows and it is very evident that he is feeling good about himself.

Loving and accepting a child who has drained and given little in return to his parents is a tough assignment, but the rewards are coming now for the first time in six years.

We *are* finding Tim desirable and loving. He wants to please. We believe that if we keep the picture of a happy, warm little boy in our minds at all times, this is exactly the way he will become.

We think one never comes to a place where he feels totally effective in handling a hyperactive child, but each day, each week, each year, we get closer. Psychologically this helps us survive.

JAMIE

It is especially important to know that the Jamie who hits the home run to start this story is not only hyperactive but also suffers from cerebral palsy (spastic hemiplegia). His mother has related a story that shows tremendous bravery (in addition to an understanding beyond belief) on the part of the entire family. The two other children in the family offer help not only to Jamie but to their parents, who had the advantage of knowing what "Normal" children were like—unlike so many of the parents in the other stories. Jamie's story is one of accomplishment—through hard work and sacrifice on everyone's part.

"I made a home run, Mommy. I did it!" He throws his arms around my neck and plants a big happy kiss on my cheek. His eyes sparkle with excitement and at that moment he is feeling the enormous sense of achievement that belongs to all small boys who hit that first home run. His dad grins at him like the proudest coach on earth; then his eyes meet mine and for a split second we share a victory that can only be understood by parents of a handicapped child. Jamie interrupts our reverie by tugging at his father's hand and impatiently reminding him that "we have to play ball some more!"

As I watch them I am struck once again by the sense of

confidence that Alex is always able to impart to Jamie. He carefully controls his movements to fit Jamie's, which are not coordinated. The ball is delivered with such slow precision that it is almost certain to hit the bat when Jamie swings. Jamie wins this way and the winning will give him courage to keep trying when the ball game gets tougher.

Later Alex and I sit on the patio absorbed in our own thoughts while Jamie plays in his sandbox with a friend. Alex smiles and reaches for my hand. "He is so special...did you see how proud he was when he hit the ball!" We sit quietly, sharing without words the joy that is Jamie's gift to us. Our marriage was good before Jamie, and sharing in his growing has brought us even closer together. This child has taught us so much about loving and has made us grow far beyond our own limitations. Temporal values are rapidly discarded and your living assumes a deeper purpose when you are sharing in a child's struggle to surmount a handicap.

Jamie is six years old and he has an older sister and brother. Jamie's story is really their story too, for they have loved him so completely and taught him with unlimited patience. From the beginning they seemed to understand with their hearts that which was far too complex for them to grasp intellectually. As the years have gone by they have each found a special relationship with Jamie. Joe has grown from a broken-hearted seven-year-old boy who sat at the kitchen table crying angrily, "But it isn't fair—I don't want my brother to be brain damaged," to a twelve-year-old big brother in every sense of the word who has learned that you can be hurt and still carry on. Ruth, at nine, lacks Joe's comprehension and has more of a whimsical nature. Joe is the one who crawled on his knees for days behind Jamie's trike teaching him how to pedal; after several pairs of worn-out jeans Joe's determination paid off, and when Jamie finally pedaled that tricycle Joe was ecstatic. Ruth never appears to see any of Jamie's deficits, nor does she want to talk about it. She just cuddles him in her own quiet way. If she goes to a party, there is always something in her pocket for Jamie when she comes home. She is the one who includes him in on a puppet show or lemonade stand and leads him through a social adventure with the assumption that he can do anything she can do! Together they have given Jamie the skills that make it possible for him to be part of that special world that belongs to all children and can never be taught by adults.

Jamie's story really begins during the first trimester of my pregnancy. He was an Rh baby, and in addition I had a placental deficiency which disrupted normal fetal development. The pregnancy was difficult, and frequent blood counts indicated that the Rh antibody count was rising to a deleterious level. A placental separation during delivery increased Jamie's trauma. At birth his respiration and reflexes were very depressed and he was jaundiced. He was immediately placed in an incubator in the intensive care unit. Alex saw him for only the few seconds that it took to switch his incubator from the delivery room to the premature nursery. He remembers racing down the hall behind Jamie's incubator frantically trying to see him and then suddenly realizing that Jamie was in severe distress. There were no answers for Alex—everyone was too busy with Jamie.

I was heavily sedated for the first twenty-four hours and can still remember waking occasionally and trying to reach through the haze of medication to ask for Jamie. I will always remember Alex sitting beside my bed with tears streaming down his face when he thought that I was asleep. When I finally did awaken there were all sorts of flowers for me and one tiny bouquet set apart from all the others. That one belonged to Jamie and the card said, "I love you very much, Jamie...Daddy."

Those first days were rather like being suspended in time and space. Jamie was fighting to live somewhere down the hall and I was not allowed to see him. A blood transfer had been performed because of the high antibody level and he was being kept under ultraviolet light to arrest the progression of the disease, which ravaged his blood system and threatened further destruction of his entire system. Rh babies can sustain brain damage as well as impairment of heart and liver function. Initially our only concern was that he live. The question of normalcy had not reached a level of consciousness for us at that point.

As Jamie improved and the time to take him home drew near, my fears began to surface. His body seemed drawn on one side and he still had difficulty with breathing and nursing. I had been taught how to aspirate his bronchial tubes and throat to clear out the persistent accumulation of mucous that he was unable to expel on his own. His pediatrician assured me that everything was going to be fine. "Just take him home and love him, we'll take care of everything as it comes."

But taking Jamie home was not that simple. He couldn't nurse without frequent choking episodes and he would often tire after only an ounce or so. His face would become contorted with a telltale blueness around the lips after only a short period of sucking. We were advised to use preemie nipples and to enlarge the holes to make it easier for him, but even this modification did not fully solve the problem. The only solution for the first few weeks was to feed him a small amount each hour or so. Within two weeks after we had brought him home he developed a massive bronchial infection and began running a high fever. This was to become a chronic pattern for him during the next two years. He was switched from one antibiotic to another, since we could barely get one infection under control before he began another. He had pneumonia twice during that first year; the pediatrician finally decided that the only thing to do was to keep him in one room that could be sterilized daily and properly filtered and humidified. In order to keep Jamie with us he had to be isolated; maintaining a hospital room in a home is not easy. This was probably the most difficult experience that Alex and I had ever had to face. We made it through that year, but it was not an optimal situation for Jamie or anyone else in the family.

I have discussed this aspect of Jamie's development because it is not unusual for neurologically impaired children to be extremely susceptible to illness during the first year. Throughout that first year Jamie's developmental delay was becoming more apparent, but the excuse was always that he had been sick a lot and would catch up later. From the beginning he had kept his left hand clutched tightly with his fist drawn up across his chest. His head was pulled over to one side and almost rested on his shoulder and his left leg was rigid and extended most of the time. By the time Jamie was six months old the pediatrician would not really look at me when he examined Jamie, but he would hold Jamie in his arms and touch him with such pain in his eyes that I knew something was very wrong. I knew also that this man who had cared for children for thirty years could not bring himself to say the words.

Once when Jamie was nine months old and I thought that I could not stand not knowing any longer, I blurted out the fear that had been slowly tearing me apart. He is brain-damaged, isn't he? Please tell me something." The doctor slowly dressed Jamie and then walked over to the window with the baby in his arms. He could not answer my question. Instead, he gazed out of the window and replied in a barely audible voice, "It is such a beautiful day that Jamie should be able to be outdoors for a short while perhaps. He is such a fine boy." This doctor *never* did manage to acknowledge there was a problem.

It isn't easy to play God; the words are hard to say when you love children. Often parents are angry when doctors fail to tell them that their child is significantly delayed in development. As a parent of a brain-damaged child I understand what it feels like to be afraid for your child and to find no answers, but I also understand why it is difficult for a doctor to take that step when there is little hope that a child might catch up. The philosophy about waiting until a developmentally delayed child is older to finally discuss the prognosis tends to be based on the assumption that the parents will have established a more spontaneous and normal relationship with the child. In reality the problem with procrastinating is that most parents cannot effectively deal with the gnawing fear, which has a subtle erosive effect on their emotions. Delaying the necessary confrontation of a problem usually results in building a defense system derived from a curious mixture of denial, anger, fear, and guilt. A parent thrust into a highly emotional state for a prolonged period of time will inevitably project this to the child. The tension and anxiety resulting from not fully comprehending a child's disability may be far more damaging than early confrontation and appropriate counseling, which can enable a parent to cope more adequately with his child's needs.

Knowing what was wrong with Jamie was not going to change the problem, but it was something that had to be faced so that we could find a peace within ourselves as parents and begin to create the appropriate atmosphere for Jamie's growing. I can remember our enormous frustration in not knowing what to do for Jamie or what to expect. Early in his infancy he began to show signs of severe hyperactivity. He cried incessantly for hours each day, and holding him only made it worse. When he was one year of age he began pounding his head violently against the headboard of his crib. He would thrash and scream if we picked him up; when I put him back in his crib he would resume his mechanical rhythmic head pounding, which could last for hours. He was closing the door on us and retreating into a strange world that frightened me. Eye contact was minimal; he would look past us and fixate on some object within his range of vision. We determined then that we would not allow him to retreat into a pattern of self-stimulation that could supersede his exploration of the world around him. We touched him constantly and talked and turned his face towards ours. The playpen had nothing to offer a child like Jamie; we kept him on the floor for the most part, which encouraged him to try to crawl and to reach for things. We worked diligently to improve the responsiveness of his spastic left side by placing objects to the left so that he would be inclined to reach with that arm. We always reinforced the use of his left hand by opening the hand and helping him to grasp whatever treat was being offered, such as a cookie or small toy. Gradually his fist unfurled and he began to use that arm and hand, no longer holding it clenched against his chest. The same progress occurred with his leg as he became more adept at crawling. Crawling was no small feat for Jamie, and it did not occur spontaneously. Initially he could manage only a weak, fishtail lunging, which didn't propel him very far. As cruel as it seemed to a few of our well-intended neighbors, I spent the better part of one summer carrying him to the edge of our backyard and then walking away from him towards the house. The object of course was to make Jamie crawl to me. This was not easy for Jamie or for me, but it had to happen if he was to gain strength in his legs. At first I would position myself only a few feet away and then kneel down on the grass and coax him. He cried many tears of frustration, but slowly he managed to crawl increasingly longer distances. The soft texture of the lawn actually aided in his gripping capacity; a carpet would have served the same purpose. I might add that there was always an abundance of hugging and kissing as well as a small treat, like a cookie when he finished his exercise. As tough as it may be to force independence when your child is damaged, the rewards for the child are what parenthood is all about.

We moved to a large city shortly after Jamie's first birthday. I carefully selected a new pediatrician, realizing that the time had come to seek a full evaluation of Jamie's problem. The new doctor confirmed Jamie's developmental delay and the apparent spasticity on his left side. By eighteen months Jamie was walking and even running, but in a very awkward fashion. New problems were evolving as he matured. He had become so hyperactive that he was sleeping only three to four hours per night. His head pounding had increased in degree and duration; he was pounding several hours a day on the floor or against the walls, in addition to his usual nighttime episodes. A resultant self-inflicted concussion made it necessary for him to be fitted with a protective padded helmet, which he wore at all times. He was beginning to compulsively repeat activities such as opening and closing a door over and over unless you stopped him and managed to redirect his attention to something else. He was not playing with toys at all, but simply running like a wild thing all day long. He would grab at anything in his path, throw it, and go on to something else. Mealtimes were extremely difficult for him because he could not sit still in his high chair long enough to eat. His impulsivity resulted in food thrown to the floor and violent temper tantrums as he struggled to climb out of his chair. He had to be watched constantly because he had no apparent sense of danger. Once he knocked the screen out of an upstairs window and was climbing out when we caught him just in time. Another time he grabbed hot charcoal out of the grill and burned his hand badly. Jamie was not able to learn from the experience. A week later he made a beeline for the grill and would have repeated the incident if his father had not grabbed his hand in time.

As Jamie became more reckless and driven like a whirling demon, the strain was beginning to show on the entire family. Alex and I were constantly on guard, and one of us had to be trailing Jamie all the time. Alex's job required a fair amount of travel; there were weeks when I was so tired from days of having only a few hours sleep that when Alex returned he would have to take over. The children were trying to understand and to cope, but the stress and strain had become almost too great for them to handle. Life for Jamie and for each of us had become a sort of nightmarish experience, which can only be described as living within the eye of a tornado.

Fortunately help was at hand. Our new pediatrician had decided to refer Jamie to a neurologist. He made the appointment for us and tried to prepare me by saying, "It doesn't look very good for Jamie right now, but let's see what can be done for him."

It is funny how we search for the truth and yet sometimes really dread finding it. As we sat in the neurologist's waiting room, Alex and I took turns trying to keep Jamie from overturning lamps and tables or shredding the magazines into a million pieces. Within a few minutes his crisp blue sunsuit was soaked with perspiration and one strap was dangling where he had torn off the button. Jamie could not tolerate confinement for even a short length of time; by the time the nurse appeared to tell us that the doctor was ready for us, Jamie was rolling around on the floor, pounding his head, and sobbing. Alex picked him up and carried him screaming and kicking into the examination room.

We had been told that this neurologist had a special gift with damaged children; we found that to be an understatement. She sat down on the floor and asked Alex to put Jamie down beside her. Jamie began running back and forth to the door, crying and pounding his head like a frightened, trapped animal. She began to softly say his name repeatedly and slowly he edged toward her. She began showing him various toys to see what he could do, and I was painfully aware that she was progressively dropping down to an infant level of task performance. It was impossible to gain Jamie's attention for more than a few seconds. As she began undressing him, Jamie lunged off the table headfirst and we barely managed to break his fall. She returned to the floor with him, wrestled him into a firm grip, and held him tightly until he stopped fighting. She then completed the undressing, stroking his back softly and talking to him soothingly until he finally relaxed. She went over his body slowly, checking reflexes, noting subtle structural abnormalties and the spasticity on the left side.

When she finished she turned to us and said very gently, but firmly, "Jamie is brain-damaged and will need a great deal of help. We will need an EEG and other tests, but I feel certain that medication will help control the hyperactivity."

There was a terrible silence for a few minutes, broken only by Jamie's jabbering to himself as he resumed running back and forth between the door and opposite wall. Alex stared at the floor fighting back the tears. I found myself floating on the edge of reality. It was as though this were happening to someone else. I heard myself asking in a strangled whisper, "Is he retarded?" For the first time during the evaluation this beautiful doctor allowed herself to express emotion. She looked at us with tears brimming in her eyes and answered, "I cannot be sure in terms of degree; we will have to perform psychological tests. But Jamie is approximately one year behind in development, which represents a significant delay at two years old. To answer your question, Jamie appears to be retarded."

You are never ready to hear these words, no matter how important it may be in the long run. I remember thinking, "I cannot stand this, it hurts too much." Alex knew that I was too devastated to be able to say anything else and he took over. "What can we do for him?" She then told us about various special developmental programs for neurologically impaired children in our community, but reminded us that we could only take a step at a time. As we left she said, "The main thing now is to complete his tests and try a medication program. If we can get the hyperactivity under control, we may be able to reach him and teach him."

A week or so later the tests were completed and the medication program was begun. Jamie responded well to the initial dosage and began to stabilize as the dosage was slowly brought up to the proper level. Medication is not the answer for all hyperactive children, but for Jamie it has provided an opportunity for development. His medication must be monitored carefully and it has been changed at various times. Without medication he was locked into a world that he could not escape from. He was so unable to cope with his environment that he had no choice but to try to run away from it. The head pounding reflected the frenzy of a child fairly exploding with an overflow of stimulation that his neurological system could not filter or effectively process. Eventually the head pounding turned into convulsant seizures. The addition of anticonvulsant therapy to his medication program has brought the seizures under relatively good control. There are no magic cures, but appropriate medication maintenance has enabled Jamie to maximize his developmental potential. Once he was calmed down, we could begin working with him more effectively. It is important to remember, however, that even when a physician elects to prescribe medication for a neurologically impaired child, the improvement must be recorded in terms of relativity. A treatment program may slow the hyperactive central nervous system to more functional limits, but the acquisition of satisfactory behavior control must occur through a learning process. While children with organically based behavior disorder may significantly respond to medication in terms of reducing the overwhelming degree of hyperactivity, they will still remain impulsive, restless, and distractible to varying degrees. The concept of medication is not to totally sedate or tranquilize a child into passive oblivion, but to simply increase his awareness and attention span to an optimal level that will hopefully allow him to respond more appropriately and develop self-control. If there are accompanying physical deficits like Jamie's spasticity and spinal curvature or if specific intellectual limitations exist, then they must be taken into consideration as part of the overall development potential. These deficits must be accepted and worked with accordingly.

Jamie fits the pattern of a learning disabled child more than that of frank retardation. His overall intellectual capacity is within low normal limits according to current psychological testing at age six. Obviously he has made a lot of progress. The important thing for him and for us as his parents is to be able to rejoice in his progress while always remembering that his abilities are scattered. For example, Jamie's verbal ability is good both receptively and expressively. He can conceptualize and problem solve effectively under structured conditions. His coordination for fine motor tasks is very poor; at six he really has to struggle to hold a pencil and can control it only well enough to copy a simple design. Integration of certain visual tasks is difficult for him and he tends to be perceptually disordered. Consequently reading and writing, particularly, will represent areas of difficulty. Jamie's attention span is extremely short and his frustration tolerance is quite limited. So when we say that Jamie tests within normal limits intellectually, that really does not mean much unless we are able to understand that capacity and performance are two separate areas. Jamie was obviously a bright child inherently, prior to the prenatal conditions that resulted in his defects. Perhaps for this reason he has been able to sustain substantial neurological impairment and still function within as high a range as he does. But we never delude ourselves as parents into recording the progress he has made without remembering the enormous amount of effort and length of time that has produced that.

In order for Jamie to have reached what his psychologist terms an optimal level of development in relationship to his neurological damage, he has had to work very hard each day in a structured rehabilitation program. Jamie has been in a developmental program for brain-damaged children for three years. He is in school from 9:00 to 2:30 everyday, which means that he has logged a lot of hours of language and physical therapy, behavior shaping, and direct academic teaching. His program is carefully structured to meet his developmental needs; he has progressed from the nursery school level to a kindergarten sequence that will last until he is seven. Eventually Jamie will pass this program and be placed into a special classroom for neurologically handicapped children within the public school system.

The strength of Jamie's program is that he has been able to share a world that is just right for him with other children who have similar problems. But even the most comprehensive rehabilitation program will fail if the child is not adequately supported by his family. Jamie's self-esteem is as high as the sky. He has been allowed to grow at a pace that is right for him. His disruptive behavior is worked with constantly within boundaries that he can fully understand, but the behavior is never confused with the child. We might not like what he is doing at the moment and he is frequently faced with the logical consequences of an inappropriate behavior, but he has never been rejected as a person. The behavior is always separated out from Jamie as a wholly loved and accepted family member. This separation is imperative, I think, if you are to successfully parent a child with behavior disorder.

Winning is especially important for a child like Jamie. This requires parents to work very hard to make certain that winning occurs more frequently than losing. It isn't easy to be a brain-damaged or hyperactive child. You cannot sit still or concentrate for more than a few moments, your body is clumsy and will not do what you want it to do, it is tough to learn things that are simple for most children, and you have to keep on trying when sometimes you would like to just give up. Winning happens when the people around you understand and fit their steps to yours.

Jamie feels good about himself. He is eager to learn and proud of all that he can do. In the process of building his self-esteem we have acquired a great deal of patience and understanding. These qualities are essential if you are to succeed in building a world that is right for a damaged child.

We were fortunate in locating doctors and psychologists who were willing to help us understand what Jamie's world was really like. It was apparent that he had been assaulted by an overload of stimuli that he could not handle. We began by literally stripping the house, especially his room, of unnecessary clutter and confusion. I worked with him for short intervals in his room, which was basically empty except for his bed, dresser, and a small table. He could sit for short periods at that table facing me for language lessons. His vocabulary was carefully expanded from a base of a few concrete words. As a new word was added, he always had the object or a picture of the object present with the word. We went from nouns to simple verbs and then to descriptive words or adjectives. At three his vocabulary was fairly extensive, but his sentences had a peculiar mechanical sound. This is a common early language pattern in brain-damaged children. They tend to learn repetitive phrases as discrete units long before they are capable of generating creative language. Providing a strong language foundation is most important; spontaneity will emerge later.

As difficult as it was at times, we required Jamie to verbalize for everything he wanted. Gestures or whining were not adequate; we would hold the cookie, for example, until he finally offered a verbal approximation of that word. Language therapy must be fun and highly reinforcing for a child with expressive language disability. Consequently, every effort that Jamie made at speaking was enthusiastically praised and rewarded. Gradually we shaped more complex language patterns for him by labeling everything in his environment and consistently talking in short sentences about whatever he was doing or we were doing. This approach was continued by his speech therapist when he entered the developmental program a year later at age three. It is hard to believe that the six-year-old magpie who talks constantly now and whose language facility is his strongest asset was originally diagnosed as a child with significant expressive language disorder.

Motor development has followed a similar pattern, although the degree of improvement has not been as great as hoped for. We began by introducing simple fine motor tasks such as large blocks for stacking, a jumbo pegboard, large beads for stringing, simple puzzles, and fat crayons or books for coloring and drawing. He has spent many happy hours at the kitchen sink filling containers and pouring water, painting at an easel with fat brushes that are easy to hold, and pounding nails with an oversized hammer. Outdoor play has been his refuge, for there he can be truly free. He loves the sandbox, jungle gym, and most of all his tree house, which has both a ladder and rope for climbing. We encourage bike riding, swimming, and ball play on a regular basis; in the winter he swims at the local YMCA, which has a heated pool. This summer he learned how to jump from the diving board and swim to the side of the pool. When he climbed out of the pool after the first big dive, his eyes shining with pride and a smile like sunshine lighting his face, our whole family cheered like crazy and admittedly had to wipe away a few proud tears of our own.

Jamie's orthopedist laughs and says, "Jamie is the only six-year-old spastic hemiplegic kid I know who can skate, ride a bike, and swim!" Jamie wears a built-up shoe to compensate for an underdeveloped leg and uses a special device attached to his pencil to enable him to grasp it well enough to write. But the important thing is that instead of psychologically separating the damaged portion of his body, he has learned to make it work for him.

In terms of behavioral development, the battle has been slow for Jamie. He is still highly excitable and cannot cope well with new situations or confusion. We learned several years ago that we can act as buffers when the world is simply too much for him to handle. Even now, I watch him closely for signs of fatigue or stress; it is much better to intervene before he falls apart than to wait until he is climbing the walls. He requires a fairly consistent routine and needs to know what to expect each day. Only recently has he reached the point where he can benefit from and enjoy social activities that involve larger groups of children. When he was younger we did not take him to the zoo, crowded stores, birthday parties, or any of the other places that are usually such fun for children. By reducing his daily level of environmental stimulation to a minimal level and then gradually introducing new experiences over the past four years, we have provided the opportunity for him to acquire skills adequate enough to allow him to cope with a moderate amount of stress or excitement at his present age. Jamie is a barometer of environmental pressure; when he begins to become overly excited and irritable, we know that it is time to slow everything down for him.

If hyperactive children share one trait in common, it is that they become rapidly more excited as they lose control and more out of control as they become excited. It is a vicious spiral plunging the hyperactive child into a frenzy of impulsive activity that can result only in increasing frustration and negative feedback. For the hyperactive child out of control, it is imperative for his parents to be in control. Good control is not won through abusive punishment or by parents who lose control of their own emotions. Control means being able to be objective, rational, and decisive in doing whatever is best for your child with a minimal amount of delay and talking. A tantrum should mean that the child is either completely ignored or led quietly to his room, picked up and carried there if necessary, to stay relatively isolated until the tantrum is over. Few words are necessary or useful when a child is in the process of exploding. "Time out" periods allow the child to cry or kick or do whatever he must do to release his rage in the privacy of his own room without having that reinforced by reactions of his parents. When the child is quiet and ready to rejoin his family, the episode is really over and he needs to be praised lovingly for having a happy face again or whatever expression may suit the situation.

Jamie learned long ago that there are no shades of gray. Our guidelines tend to be absolute in terms of behavioral expectations. We try to avoid unnecessary demands and to allow him as much behavioral freedom as possible. We try to be flexible in terms of the stress level he may be experiencing under certain conditions. He hears "no" very seldom, but when we say it we mean it. We think carefully before we ask any task of him, because once we do, he is expected to follow through. Consequently, Jamie has learned to work well within consistent behavioral parameters and a large measure of his security seems based on the fact that he is not faced with needless conflicts about what is acceptable and what is not. Teaching Jamie acceptable social behavior is just as important as any other therapy in his rehabilitation program, because the mastery of social skills will largely determine how well he can be integrated into society as he matures.

The most important gift that a parent can bestow upon any child, whether he is normal or handicapped, is complete acceptance of that child as an individual. Jamie is special not because he is handicapped, but simply because he is Jamie. His life must have purpose and he must be free to reach for everything that is important to him. The promise of his tomorrow will be secured by his belief in himself. He does not comprehend quitting and understands little about losing, because he sees himself as a winner. He wins simply by trying and he knows that. I am reminded of a race he ran last year against several neighborhood children who were far more fleet than he. He stayed behind all of the others but doggedly continued on to the finish line; he rolled over on the grass in a happy heap and grinned up at me and said, "I ran fast Mommy...I won too!" He did not beat the other children; he was not competing against them, Jamie was simply running with them and competing only against himself. He understands, I think, that all that really matters is that you do your very best. Someday he will learn all about losing and he may be hurt along the way, but I believe that he will be so secure within himself that he will be strong enough to keep reaching for the victories that can be his.

Perhaps Jamie's story sounds too perfect or unrealistically happy, but we do not sing sad songs. Jamie has brought great joy to his family and we have all grown more complete as individuals. Sharing Jamie's enthusiasm for life and his abundant willingness to work so hard to achieve has taught each of us how to use his own gifts more fully. Jamie carries on a love affair with the world that has an almost charismatic quality. Everyone he meets responds to his smile and he has more friends than we could probably begin to count. He has taught a great many people about the meaning of loving and sharing and I like to think that he has helped to carve a pathway of understanding for other brain-damaged children who are asking simply to be helped to grow in ways that are right for them and to be free to share the world that belongs to all children.

DANIEL

There are two items that especially set off Daniel's story from the rest. He is an extremely bright child, a factor that is not especially typical of hyperactive children, and he is now thirteen years old. None of the other children in these stories is near that age. We can follow the progress of Daniel's development and that of his parents who contributed so much. While it is notable that Daniel has no *learning difficulties, one of his primary deficiencies is his social problems. He also has poor coordination. At the time his problems began to manifest themselves, it was not as easy to find help as it is now. He has a younger sister, now ten.*

Our first child, a son, was born in the summer of 1963. Delivery was normal, and it was a very happy occasion for us.

Other than a milk allergy, all went well during the first few months. The baby thrived on Probana, a banana-based formula. He seemed bright and alert and followed a fairly routine eating and sleeping schedule.

But his large motor development seemed slow. By this we mean that he was late in pulling himself up to a chair and was late to sit up unsupported. He did not walk alone until fourteen months. He never crawled at all.

From about eight months he enjoyed bouncing in a spring-suspended jumper. He enjoyed this so much that he twice wore out the vinyl sling-type seat and it had to be replaced.

Shortly after his first year he was ill with a high fever. A blood test showed it to be a viral infection. The pediatrician suspected roseola, but the rash never appeared. In a few days he was better.

Toys did not seem to interest him very much. Once he had examined one and tested a toy, he lost interest and threw it aside.

When he began to navigate on his own, he would dash to and fro opening cupboards, pulling books out of bookcases, emptying drawers, and grabbing anything he could get his hands on. No amount of reasoning, cajoling, or spanking could get him to willingly stop something we disapproved of. He was very determined to get what he wanted. His attention span was extremely short; he would flit from one thing to another. His determination and absorption made him oblivious to everyone around him.

The only exception to this seemed to be when we read to him. Then he would sit and listen, and as he grew older he enjoyed hearing the same stories over and over again. He was also fascinated by water and took great delight in mixing together water, detergents, and any other liquids he could get his hands on.

While his frantic dashing about irritated and frustrated us, we did not feel at the time that he was abnormal. We merely assumed that all children were like this.

The times that were the most difficult for us were when we took him with us to the homes of friends and relatives. At these times he was especially active. He would not sit still for a moment. He frantically dashed about opening closets and drawers, turning on appliances, running water, and getting into all kinds of mischief.

His behavior was trying and embarrassing for us. No matter what we did in the way of advance planning (bringing along new toys, etc.), nothing worked. As we look back now, he seemed to be completely disoriented by the strange surroundings, and he expressed his confusion by staying in perpetual motion.

He had as a small child, and continued to have as he grew older, a very negative attitude. What he wanted almost always was the opposite of what those around him wanted. He seemed like the round peg in the square hole.

Once when he was about three and a half, I left him with a friend who had a child his age and two younger children. When I returned to pick him up she greeted me at the door with, "I took him this time, but please don't ever ask me again!"

Needless to say, I never did ask any other friend to take him. It was at times like these that I experienced a real sense of failure—a feeling that I had done or was doing something wrong that caused him to be the way he was. Taking him shopping or visiting was often a humiliating experience because I felt that everyone believed his behavior was my fault.

The time when we really began to feel that something was wrong was when he started nursery school shortly after his third birthday. It was a large laboratory school associated with a state university. The physical plant was large and so was the number of children enrolled. As we look back on it now and see things in perspective, this situation was the worst possible one we could have chosen for him.

He was a complete misfit. He had nothing whatever to do with the other children except when they tried to interfere with what he was doing. Then he would fight, scream, or cry.

He was totally confused and disoriented. He would rush in each day and immediately head for the easel and paints. Then he would take all the open cans of paint and dump them into the water pail. When he did communicate with others, it was with the adults, not the children.

His coordination was poor. He was very apprehensive about going up and down stairs. For several years (up until the time he was six or seven) he walked up and down stairs a step at a time, placing both feet on each step before proceeding to the next one.

The child was extremely verbal. He talked constantly whether or not anyone was listening.

For his third birthday he received a tricycle. He sat on it and enjoyed ringing the bell, but he showed little interest in riding it. We showed him how to pedal, but after going a few feet he would quit.

We also had a swing in our yard, but he shied away from the conventional wooden seat. He was afraid to balance on it. Instead he preferred to sit in the glider, which had a back support and foot rest. He would sit in this, and we would push him back and forth.

We also purchased a jungle gym with ladders and bars, hoping he would become interested in climbing and overcome some of his fear of high places. But he showed little interest. He would climb as far as the first rung and then quit.

Of all the toys he ever had, the two that gave him the most pleasure were a rocking horse (suspended on springs) and a phonograph. These together gave him hundreds of hours of entertainment. He would rock on the horse in time to the music—the faster, the better. He received the horse when he was three years old and he rocked and rocked until finally he grew too large for it. This was when he was about seven or eight.

When he was two, he began having strep infections which led to ear infections and hearing problems.

Unfortunately, these intensified when he started nursery school, and this probably contributed a great deal to his sense of confusion. We were not always aware of the fact that his ears were so filled with fluid that he was unable to hear properly. Finally, when he was three and a half he had his tonsils and adenoids removed. This improved his ear problems considerably, although he still suffered from occasional strep infections.

Our second child, a daughter, was born in late 1966. She had colic very badly and cried day and night for the first few months. This put a strain on all of us. We had done our best to prepare our son for the baby's arrival and kept assuring him that we still loved him even after the new baby arrived. But during this time he began to experience nightmares. He would cry out in his sleep, but it was difficult to wake him and almost always impossible to fathom what he had been dreaming. This continued off and on for several months and eventually he stopped having the nightmares.

While our pediatricians were always good at treating his infections, they were very little help as far as his other problems were concerned. Whenever we tried to bring up the subject of his poor coordination and his extreme physical activity, they responded with shrugs or brushoffs like, "Don't worry about it."

They could easily shrug it off, but we had to live with it day after day, week after week. We knew we needed help. Finally, my husband phoned our pediatrician and insisted that he refer us to someone who could help us. He gave us the name of a pediatric neurologist at the city's children's hospital.

The neurologist gave our son various tests and confirmed that he was hyperactive. She categorized him as having "minimal brain dysfunction," and prescribed medication on a trial basis. After trying Ritalin and Dexadrine with unsuccessful results, we settled on Mellaril. This drug seemed to calm him down somewhat, but we continued to have many of the same problems.

A few months before the boy's fifth birthday my husband accepted a new position, and we moved to another state. Our new neighborhood had several children our son's age, but he still had difficulty making friends or playing peacefully. When he did play, it was primarily with girls. Because of his poor coordination girls were probably less of a threat to him.

He got through kindergarten without too much difficulty. At least, we heard very few complaints from the teacher. I guess we assumed at this point that "no news was good news," so we decided to leave well enough alone.

But he was having problems walking to and from school. Many times he was pushed around and ridiculed by older boys. It was some time before we were able to fit all the pieces together, because he did not tell us in the beginning about what was going on. We discussed the problem with the school principal, who was a kindly older woman, and she rectified the problem. She found out who the troublemakers were and put a stop to it.

His school years have been filled with teasing and ridicule. Because of his poor coordination, he has often been called a "fairy" and told that he was "queer." Also, his tendency to overreact makes him a sitting duck for teasing. Other children soon become aware that they can get his goat, and he falls right into their traps.

There were times, though, when he seemed to be really asking for trouble. At home he was continually testing the rules, always looking for loopholes and pushing as far as he could. He was determined to get his own way even if it meant flirting with disaster. At times he was like a moth circling a flame. He never seemed to know when to quit, never seemed to know when to leave well enough alone.

He is extremely intelligent. He learned reading, as well as all of his other academic subjects, easily and well. If he does have a specific learning disability, it is a handicap involving his social relationships. He has difficulty picking up social cues from other people, difficulty realizing when someone is annoyed or upset. As a young child he did not respond to quiet words or gentle actions, only to shouts or physical restraint or spanking. There were times when we felt like beating him to a pulp! (But fortunately, we never did.)

Because he was so bright and so verbal, it was easy at times to forget that he was just a child. Sometimes I would look at him lying asleep in his bed, and the realization that he was just a child would hit me, and I would feel very guilty about how angry I had become with him during the course of the day.

When he was about six we again took him to a pediatric neurologist for a reevaluation. She had us ease him off the Mellaril, with the intention of trying him on a new drug. But after he was off the Mellaril we felt that he really wasn't very different from the way he had been when he was on it. So my husband and I made the decision to keep him off drugs completely.

All during the months that our son had been on medication, my husband and I had disagreed about it. He felt we should be giving him the maximum dosage that the neurologist had told us was safe. But I had serious doubts because I feared the child might suffer side effects from prolonged use of the drug which might not manifest themselves for several years. So I was relieved when he was taken off the medication.

It was about this time that we had a physical therapist work with him individually to try to improve his coordination. She saw him once a week and taught him various exercises which he was supposed to practice each day. This continued for a couple of months, but he became so uncooperative about practicing that we finally just gave up. The negative effects far outweighed the positive, if indeed there were any positive ones.

When he was about seven years old we sought help at a

child guidance clinic run by the psychology department of a state university. This involved testing the child and extensive interviews and discussions between us and members of the psychology staff. It also involved our son being in a play therapy group with three or four other children. Our association with the clinic lasted about two years, up until the time we again moved to another state.

I don't feel we gained a great deal of help from the clinic. Our son seemed to benefit least of all. My husband and I probably gained some insights into our family relationships through the interviews and discussions, but not really enough to make it all seem worthwhile.

In second grade our boy had a teacher who disliked him intensely. She was quite old and suffered from severe arthritis, and he was more than she could tolerate. The result was that both she and our son were very miserable. We had to work fairly hard to accomplish it, but we did succeed in getting him transferred to another school in the same district. He was much happier there, and the following year he returned to his old school.

At the time we moved our son had just completed the third grade. A new home in a new city meant starting all over again. We always held out hope that a fresh start for him might be a good thing. But unfortunately, many of our old problems moved right along with us. It didn't take long for him to be labelled and zeroed in on by other children. His chip-on-the-shoulder attitude, his tendency to overreact and burst into tears, his poor coordination, all drew attention. At times we compared him to a bull fighter waving a red cape, inviting confrontation.

He attended public school through the fourth grade. While he continued to do well academically, he was very unhappy. It was a struggle just getting him to go to school each day. His social relationships were far from satisfying and much of the time he was bored because there was little in the way of academic challenge. This all added up to problems and more unhappiness for him and for our whole family.

There was never any doubt in our minds that he was very intelligent. Both my husband and I are professional educators, and our son's observations told us that he was bright and gifted. Our opinions were confirmed by standardized achievement tests that were administered in school. He consistently scored several grade levels above the norm, especially in verbal and mathematical skills.

We decided to try sending him to a private school. It meant a financial sacrifice, but we hoped it might be worth it.

About this time we again sought professional help with another pediatric neurologist. This time our son was given the most comprehensive battery of physical and mental tests he had ever received. These included everything from intelligence tests to an EEG, and even a skull Xray to check for fluid on the brain. The EEG was normal, as were all of the other medical tests. The other tests confirmed that he was exceptionally bright, but that his motor skills were poor. The doctor emphasized that the great discrepancy between his intellectual abilities and his motor skills was the cause of many of his problems and frustrations.

The doctor's initial recommendation was that we send the boy to a residential school, where a program could be tailored to his individual needs. Ideally it would be a situation geared to his unique capabilities and problems, and one in which he could succeed.

My husband and I both rejected this idea. The costs would have been more than we could afford, but even if it had been possible, there was no first-rate residential school within several hundred miles of our home. We felt that being separated from us when he was only ten years old would be too devastating. While there was no question that he continued to be a problem at home, we did love him very much and did not want him to be separated from his family.

The doctor's alternative suggestion was that we work with a child psychiatrist. This we agreed to and are continuing to do. Of all the things that we have done, this has been one of the most fruitful.

Our son is now thirteen years old and is in the eighth grade at a private school. The classes are small, and he is able to receive more individual attention. He still has bad days when he is argumentative and when he is the target for teasing by other children. He also continues to suffer from his lack of athletic prowess. Unfortunately, there is a great deal of emphasis given to athletics at his school. This bothers us because sports seem to be overemphasized.

But we feel we can't keep shuffling him from one school to another. Each move means starting all over again with many of the same problems. He is reasonably happy in his present situation. He knows everyone and they know him. He is in familiar surroundings, and he knows what to expect and what is expected of him. He continues to do well academically and seems to be making progress toward developing satisfying social relationships. He has more sensitivity to the feelings of others, and he is making strides in developing more self-control. His weekly sessions with the psychiatrist have played an important part in his progress.

At home he is becoming easier to live with, although we still have occasional bad days. When he becomes especially irritating to us we send him to his room for a cooling-off period. We set or let him set the electric range timer for anywhere from five minutes to an hour. He can come out of his room when the timer goes off. He seems to accept this, and we all benefit by it.

Sometimes when a situation arises that has the potential for causing arguments, together we draw up a written contract outlining what rules are to be followed and what penalties will result if they are not adhered to. This was the case when he received his new stereo. We outlined in advance how loud it could be played and when. If he breaks the rules, he is not allowed to play it for the next twenty-four hours.

Other disciplinary measures that we employ were depriving him of TV or fining him part of his allowance.

He seems to have outgrown much of his extreme physical activity, and his longer attention span allows him to do more constructive and satisfying things.

He has a paper route once a week and enjoys the money he earns. He is an avid reader and especially likes nonfiction. Weather is something that has interested him for several years, and he has become somewhat of an authority on the subject. Watching television and taking pictures with his pocket camera are other pastimes he enjoys.

He dislikes most sports, both as a participant and as a spectator, although he does find pleasure in bowling and table tennis. For the past three summers he has attended day camp at a local farm. The camp is very well run, and children are allowed to choose from a variety of activities with no pressure being put upon them to participate in athletics.

He has participated in the camp swim classes. And while he's made progress in overcoming his initial fear of the water and has learned to float, he still is unable to swim. He has never learned to ride a bicycle and shows no desire to learn, in spite of our coaxing.

Unfamiliar or crowded staircases sometimes make him apprehensive, especially if they are open or glass enclosed. He also refuses to use the down escalators in department stores.

Last year he flew to Florida by himself to spend a week with his grandmother. The trip was good for his self-esteem, but he was a complete wreck when he returned home. While in Florida he had eaten in restaurants most of the time and had gorged himself on things like milk shakes and french fries. (He gained about ten pounds in that week.) Also, he stayed up late watching TV and had very little sleep.

This whole incident emphasizes the fact that he still needs a considerable amount of supervision and discipline. He functions much better and is much happier when limitations are set and a familiar routine is followed. Many times he does his best to challenge the restrictions we impose, but we are convinced he really needs them.

Popular music plays an important role in his life. He listens to it whenever he can. He has a small radio which he carries around on his paper route and puts under his pillow at night. He also has a stereo in his room and listens to it almost every day. He paces back and forth in time to the music, just as he once rocked on his toy horse as a young child.

Our son has been a Boy Scout for almost two years and seems to enjoy attending the meetings. But he wants nothing whatever to do with camping out or roughing it in the woods. On one occasion he went on a twelve-mile hike, but has since vowed never to do it again.

He is very interested in consumer affairs, and several times he has written letters of complaint, which have gotten positive results. He enjoys shopping and doing price comparisons. He will go grocery shopping for us, and armed with a shopping list and pocket calculator, will seek out the bargains and do an admirable job.

He enjoys family games such as Monopoly. For the most part he can accept losing, although he is extremely competitive and tries hard to win.

He still has no close friends that he pals around with, but he does seem to get along better with more of his classmates.

His relationship with his younger sister is not always the best. In spite of her colicky beginnings, she has developed into an easygoing, bright, lovable child. Her coordination is good, and she never showed signs of being hyperactive.

I have often wondered what our lives would have been like if she had been our first child and our son had been our second. Had we had the opportunity to raise a "normal" child first, we could have proven to ourselves, as well as everyone else, that we were capable of doing it right. When a couple's first child has many problems, there is always the tendency for the parents to be blamed. Also, if our daughter had been our first, when our son came along we would have been better prepared to recognize the early warning signs that something was wrong. I realize all of this speculation is worthless, but it's something that has gone through my mind many times.

If I were to offer advice to parents of hyperactive children, I would tell you to seek out other parents of similar children. I sincerely believe that these are the only people who truly comprehend what life is like with a hyperactive child. Over the years these parents have been invaluable to use for their help and encouragement.

Also, I would tell parents to assert themselves when they feel they are right about their child. Don't be afraid to speak out to doctors, teachers, and anyone else who influences your child's life. Sometimes as parents we experience a gut feeling about what is right for our child. And if we see a situation where the child's welfare is being jeopardized, it is our responsibility to speak up and fight, if necessary, to correct matters.

From the very beginning I would establish routines for doing things. Meals, bedtime, outings should, as much as possible, follow a predictable pattern for the child.

Parents deserve to be away from their child and have free

time to themselves occasionally. Once you have found a qualified sitter or trained one to your satisfaction, try to make the task as pleasant as possible for all concerned. Before leaving the house, try to anticipate all needs and possible emergencies. And insist that the sitter follow your established routines for meals, bedtime, etc.

Try to avoid overstimulating situations where the child is likely to become disoriented and confused. Keep distractions and decision making to a minimum. Break down complicated tasks into separate, step-by-step parts for the child.

When he begins to play with other children, introduce him to them on a one-to-one basis, rather than immersing him in a group situation.

As he grows older teach him to avoid situations where there is likely to be trouble.

Encourage him to pursue new interests and help him to seek out new information, experiences, and people to help him.

Correct him when he's wrong, but praise him at every opportunity.

Help him to like himself and take pride in the things he does well.

DIANE AND BRAD

Diane and Brad are both hyperactive, but the emphasis is on Diane's story because there are so few hyperactive girls. It is much more prevalent in boys, by a factor of approximately 7:1. Diane is five (while Brad is two) so there is much more to be said about her at this point. The tremendous strain building on parents is especially evident in this story because of Diane's long tantrums. The experimentation with medication is discussed in detail here, and it is important to note that since hyperactive children respond differently to certain drugs, it is necessary to carefully monitor medication, to find that which will increase awareness, without harmful side effects. Their mother also has emphasized the prescription that now seems to offer the family the most valuable cure—love!

Diane is a bright but extremely hyperactive girl now five years old. Her greatest learning disability is her inability to attend to matters at hand—her attention span is *very* short. She also has difficulty curbing behavior—whatever she feels like doing, she does. Her lack of inhibition has created problems in social development. Additionally, Diane has some minor fine motor disability (poor pencil control) and has poor gross motor control (clumsiness and poor running ability. Her disabilities have become apparent gradually, as she has met with various stages of development.

From her first night Diane has been a happy, active child. That night she held her head erect (turtle fashion) and introduced herself to the world.

Even During her first week, it was not unusual for Diane to push with her feet in an effort to stand. Before she was three weeks old she could sit with some help; and she preferred that position to lying. At three weeks Diane could lift her head and chest off her bed elbow height, and by six weeks she could lift herself up full arm's length.

We, her parents, were delighted with her progress. Being first-time parents, we saw nothing amiss. However, friends did comment that she did not act at one month like a cuddlesome little baby. Why? Well, she was not generally content to be cradled in our arms—instead, she preferred to climb up over our shoulders or to hold our fingers and "stand."

At three months she mastered rolling over. And at four months she began trying to feed herself. She was determined to master a glass and wanted no help from Mama. Comments from friends and even from Diane's pediatrician began to come in: "She certainly is independent."

Independent indeed! She even set her own schedule. While she did sleep some during the day and throughout the night, her very favorite time of day was that period between supper at 11:00 p.m.— sometimes later (she was a late retirer.) during this time period she played, "stood," and was a real companion to her parents. We did not, at the time, consider this schedule a problem, but Diane's sleep habits were far from normal.

Between four and five months, much to her delight, Diane became more mobile. Her walker was a source of great entertainment, and Diane took off under her own power all over the house. At the same time she was trying to sit—placed in proper sitting position, she could remain that way for a long time.

At five months, crawling came into her life. She pulled her trunk around, using her forearms.

Six months was a real milestone. Diane pulled herself to a standing position for the first time and began climbing onto and into everything. Crawling on hands and knees and sitting were perfected. By six and one-half months Diane was "walking," holding onto Mama's or Daddy's hands.

Diane could stand alone by seven and one-half months, and by eight and one-half months she was walking on her own.

At that time, she was also "talking" some — Mama, Dada, dog, etc.

With her newfound independence, Diane gradually became less easy to handle. Most of the time she was quite obedient and progressed quite well. But more and more we began to notice a very definite stubborn streak.

It became almost impossible to keep Diane in her car seat. She climbed out in spite of her seat belt. Frequently this climbing was accompanied by a tantrum— if determined little Diane did not get to do what she wanted, when she wanted, a tantrum usually ensued. Meal times were also a problem. She could not sit through a meal. In fact, keeping her attention on food was almost impossible. (And this was in spite of her very good appetite—she loved all kinds of food and would eat ravenously if we followed her around and hand-fed her.) It was very difficult to keep her in her high chair—she even got loose from her seat strap. These problems were worse for Mama than for Daddy, as they generally occurred more often during Daddy's work hours. Evening and weekends she had more attention—both parents—and Diane seemed alright. Daddy, especially, could not understand the problems Mama was beginning to have.

However, by the time Diane was fifteen months old even Daddy was beginning to see the problems Mama was having. Tantrums were becoming more lengthy and more frequent. Some of the first ones Daddy had to contend with occurred in the car. Something minor would set her off; and in a car the din was very hard to take.

Generally, tantrums occurred when she became determined to do something. No amount of correction (verbal or physical) would deter her from doing something she was bound to do. Forced to stop an activity, Diane would go into a tantrum that might last up to three or four hours. (Ignoring her or putting her in her room had no effect.) Other lengthy tantrums occurred when we, her parents, were unable to determine the cause. Perhaps she became frustrated because she was unable to communicate as she desired — we do not know.

Perhaps here it is important to describe Diane's tantrums. She did not thrash about and kick her feet. Rather, she either stood or lay on the floor, stiffened, and *screamed.* Sometimes she would run about and do things like shake a mirror off a wall or pull down curtains—screaming all the while. Placing her in a room by herself served to intensify some of her tantrums. During a tantrum it was impossible to communicate with her—she did not seem to hear us. Afterward, she usually could not tell us anything that had occurred during the tantrum or why she had been screaming.

It was about this time (age fifteen months) that our pediatrician told me that Diane was hyperactive. Prior to this we had not even considered assigning that name to her behavior. All we knew was that she threw tantrums. We had no children before to compare to Diane. Indeed, we had not considered hyperactivity as a possibility. The doctor said he would prefer not to prescribe medication at such a young age unless it became absolutely necessary.

Life did not improve by our having a diagnosis. Indeed, things continued to worsen. It became impossible to do "family" things. Diane was a "dictator." We found ourselves avoiding situations that might set off a tantrum. These were things like eating out, especially at fast-food hamburger places with lots of colors, noise, and people — too much stimulation. We would go to the zoo, but only if we were sure it wasn't crowded. Too many people meant too much stimulation, and too much stimulation meant a possible tantrum.

Routine things, however, we could not avoid. Bedtime had always been late for Diane, but now it became a real hassle for us. Just keeping her attention on dressing for bed was practically impossible. She danced, ran from us, wiggled, squirmed, got out toys — she was in constant motion. Getting her to sleep was a real job. We read to her, rocked her, played music — did anything we could think of to calm and relax her. She did not sleep until absolute physical exhaustion knocked her out. Atarax, a tranquilizer, was prescribed for bedtime, but it did not help particularly and was discontinued.

Tantrums at bedtime were the rule, not the exception.

Diane was about twenty months old when Mama gave in. That day began early. After breakfast a neighbor came over at 7:30 to leave her house key. The neighbor was a particular favorite of Diane's. When the neighbor did not stay, Diane was very unhappy; a tantrum began. From that point Diane had one tantrum after another. In general, I did not know what set off the tantrums, but by three o'clock I could take no more. The tantrums had been almost unending for the entire day and I was in tears. Nothing had gotten Diane to settle down, including spanking. Finally, I spanked her so hard that she cringed when I went toward her. It is difficult to describe what went through my mind — mostly panic. This had to stop! Why was this happening? If something was not done I would be at the brink of child abuse. (We can understand how parents of hyperactive children fall into child abuse, though we don't condone it.) I called Diane's doctor and Ritalin was prescribed.

It was not long before my husband and I began to see a big improvement in Diane. We have no choice but to attribute that change to medication.

Although at twenty months Diane was saying many words, she generally seemed to talk in streaks of jibberish. Usually we were unable to understand her; and we were beginning to be concerned about her verbal skills.

Some of Diane's fine motor skills were developing. For example, she loved puzzles, placing shapes into the correct hole, stacking cups and blocks, etc. However, while she greatly enjoyed them, she was frequently frustrated in these activities. She had great difficulty keeping her attention on one puzzle or only one of anything. She wanted to do everything at once. (This frustration at not being able to do everything at once frequently brought on tantrums.)

Her short attention span was a real problem at story time. She wanted all her books read at one time, but she could not even sit still for one simple, short one. To hold her in our laps was almost impossible — she was up and down, up and down, up and down.

Then, what amazed parents we were at the change in our baby! Diane had been on Ritalin about three days when suddenly she was speaking in clear, distinct sentences (she had slowed down enough for us to understand her.) She was using up to five and six words together in sentences, and her vocabulary seemed to multiply overnight. Fantastic!

And storytime—she could sit and listen to us read to her. She still wanted a stack of books to read, but she would settle for one at a time. Sometimes she would even sit for long periods on our laps. Puzzles and other toys became more fun for her. Diane became far more contented than she had been in months.

But—Ritalin was not a miracle drug. Those long tantrums still happened; they were just somewhat less frequent.Things went generally quite well for a while; then, problems increased again. Uping Dianes dosage of Ritalin seemed to help.

However, new kinds of problems were occurring now. Diane was having problems playing with or around other children. Many long tantrums began because she could not have the toy another child was playing with. Parents of younger children with whom this happened were afraid Diane would hurt them. They did not want Diane to play with their children. Diane also frightened some children with her compulsive hugging and touching. She would do this too much and this made the children afraid of her. (All of this ceased later after she was given a drug called Dilantin.) Diane did not intimidate aggressive children.

Alone, Diane was unable to initiate really meaningful play activity. She spent hours tearing paper into smaller and smaller pieces (she said she was making ducks, etc.) Other times she would spend long periods ordering things, sometimes by color, sometimes by shape. In general she did not play with toys the way they were meant to be played with.

This is not to say that she never played with toys correctly—she merely had trouble when she was playing alone. She was able to play with things as they were meant to be if she was guided to do so.

Her high activity level seemed perpetual. In fact, we began privately and lovingly to call her our "perpetual motion machine." At the dinner table she turned somersaults in her chair, frequently falling off the edge (luckily, with no harm done). Both at the table and away, *spinning* and *dancing* were not unusual. Television was not a good babysitter at our house, since Diane could not sit still long enough for it to "sit" with her.

Besides not being able to contain her activity, we were unable to dispell her ever mounting *fears.* While some fear is normal for small children, Diane's fears were unusually big. It seemed like these fears intensified suddenly. Diane was never able to concentrate well; and when she became aware of threatening stimuli around her (barking dogs, darkness, loud noises, cars or trucks starting, and so on) she did not know what stimulus to respond to. This created the fears. She would not play in our fenced yard without Mama by her side. If, while walking down a hallway in our home, I got a bit ahead of her, Diane would scream as though terrorized. She seemed to feel she had been deserted. Screams of terror might be heard anytime she looked up and discovered Mama (or Daddy) missing from the room. There really was no explanation for this terror, as Diane was never deserted and was not even left with a sitter very often at this time. At night she wanted a light on and did not want to be left alone. Frequently one parent had to stay with her until she dropped off to sleep.

Fearfulness is not bad—neither were Diane's other behaviors, really. It was just that they were so unending that they taxed the energy of both her parents. In general, she was a very good, obedient, and affectionate child. Nevertheless, some of her activities were just not acceptable at her age level. And as parents we found ourselves unable to change those behaviors.

As she grew bigger, our job became more difficult. Diane was once again almost impossible to get in bed at night. Her larger size and greater strength made her harder to handle. It took two adults to get her into her nightgown. We actually had to hold her down and fight to get her changed, and we began really to dread those nightly tantrums of very lengthy duration.

The state of things was not great when Diane's brother was born. Diane was two years and nine months old. She wanted her new baby, but we did have the usual problems—jealousy, etc.

Baby Brad was colicky, and this certainly did not help Mama handle Diane's problems. Bedtime continued to be a *real* problem. Mealtime had never really improved. She just could not sit and eat (we frequently found ourselves hand-feeding her just to get some food down.). And Ritalin certainly did not help (depressed appetite). We also continued to have socialization problems.

Diane was unable to curb behaviors that were not acceptable—for example, touching or hugging children who did not want to be touched or hugged; "dragging" another child to her room when the child preferred not to go; running around during mealtime; "sitting" upside down in a chair, etc. Her attention span became even more a problem.She could not attend to dressing, eating, playing, sleeping, or anything else other children her age could do. She was not toilet trained.

We felt the Ritalin was no longer doing the job, and we were also seeing behavior we did not like — particularly, periods of depression. Hence, we took her completely off medication. This did not help, although depression did end. Next we tried another medication, Cylert. It was disastrous. Things became worse, not better. She continued to be aggressive with other children. During this period (not just on Cylert) Diane destroyed toys and other things, but her destructiveness did not seem deliberate.

It became obvious that we needed more advice and information. We began reading more about hyperactivity and we sought the advice of Diane's pediatrician. He suggested that we check into a special school for Diane. (Diane had, herself, expressed interest in school.)

Diane was taken off all medication and scheduled for both psychological and neurological testing. She was enrolled in a special nursery school for summer day camp. The teachers and advisory/consulting staff observed her behavior carefully. Her age was three and one-half years. The results of psychological testing were scattered, but Diane is, at least, of normal intelligence, Some fine motor problems were noticed, as well as poor gross motor control.

Neurological testing was done in late summer. The doctor felt she was definitely hyperactive. An EEG was performed. Diane was diagnosed as having subclinical seizures. The doctor explained that these were most likely occurring *very* frequently and that they probably accounted for many of the tantrums and fears. He prescribed Dilantin. We noticed improvement, but there were some problems in adjusting the dosage. The dosage was originally three 50-mg pills per day. We became aware of gradually increasing clumsiness. Finally she became ataxic—unable to stand or crawl. After blood tests and further observation the dosage was reduced to two pills per day. (We would advise all parents contemplating medication of this sort to work very carefully with doctors and other trained observers to prevent needless overdose or other problems. *Know the drug and its side effects.*) Finally, through consultation with the neurologist, Diane's pediatrician, and her teachers, we arrived at a satisfactory medication program consisting of three drugs in mild doses — Dilantin, Diamox, and Ritalin. Diane is presently taking this combination of drugs and is doing better than ever before.

Tantrums are now far fewer. And *none* is so intense and lengthy as in the past. In general, they are normal temper tantrums that might be expected in any child. There is no stiffening, and we can get through to her and calm her down.

She still has difficulty at mealtime. She cannot properly concentrate on her meals and is very easily distracted. Somersaults continue.

However, we do find Diane's activity more easily channelled into meaningful play—and she plays with other children very well now. (Parents of playmates have noted the big change in her.)

While she still wants a light at night, Diane's fears have greatly diminished.

Generally, she is much calmer and more contented. A frequent visitor to the house has said, "I used to feel a constant inner turmoil in that child, but now it's gone."

Still there are many days when that turmoil is *very* present, when Diane cannot be calm; but we are working toward helping her learn control and inhibition of undesirable behavior.

It would be impossible to explain fully how Diane's hyperactivity affects our family without interjecting, here, a few notes about her brother, Brad.

Prior to his arrival, it was not so difficult to work around Diane's problems — she was the only child and was generally adorable. Everyone "loves" Diane because she is quite affectionate and does desire to please others, especially adults.

It is certainly less easy to contend with two young children instead of one, even if there is no disability in either child. But Brad was born with his own problems. First, he had colic and allergies. It was to these that we attributed Brad's inability to sleep at night. As time passed, however, colic and allergy subsided or improved, and Brad still was awake much of the night. Lack of sleep made him a crabby baby much of the time. As he became mobile, he became extremely hard to handle. He was larger than his sister as a baby, and stronger, too. Brad was (and is) forever climbing and was constantly into things he should not be into.

About the time we enrolled Diane in her special school, we became very suspicious, as did our pediatrician, that Brad, too, might be hyperactive. He still did not sleep at night. He would awaken screaming. His sleep was restless and he frequently rocked his bed. In fact, what he actually did was take one and one-half or two hour naps throughout the twenty-four hours, with long awake times in between.

By fall, Mama was thoroughly worn down — lack of good sleep for over a year. Brad was up much of the night, and Diane was up from early morning until sometimes late at night — she has not taken naps since she was fifteen months old. The pediatrician prescribed a mild bedtime tranquilizer for Brad. It began to work and he seemed somewhat more contented during the day (less crabby). Nevertheless, he continued to be very hard to contain.

Shopping with him was unbelievable. He was out of the shopping cart or stroller quickly and began taking things off the shelf. Physical punishment was to no avail.

In fact, Brad became almost impossible to handle. Always hard to hold, he began to push away and climb out of our arms. We could not carry him or keep him in a stroller or in a shopping cart. We could not keep him in his car seat. We could not keep him in his high chair or in a regular chair. He could and would climb into and out of almost anything we put him in. Needless to say, bumps and bruises were routine.

He did not throw tantrums like his sister, but Brad was constantly crying (usually without tears). Between Diane's tantrums and Brad's crying the house was in a constant din. It took very little to set him off.

Diane did not help. She wanted to play with everything he wanted, and he wanted everything. In fact, like his sister, Brad was not content to play with one toy at a time.

We also could not read even the simplest book to him. In this area he was worse than Diane had been, as he could sit in a lap even less time than she. Brad's attention span seemed even shorter than Diane's, and he was definitely harder to manage.

By the time he was fifteen months old we decided, for our own peace, that we must do something to calm him down. First we tried coffee. He would not drink it. Then we tried caffeine tablets. They did not phase him. Finally, at seventeen and one-half months we conceded that Brad was definitely hyperactive; and the pediatrician placed him on a mild dosage of Ritalin.

Just as with his sister, we saw dramatic improvement. While he had said only a few words prior to medication, he began talking. At first it was merely a rapidly increasing vocabulary; but by the time he had been on medication for six weeks, he was grouping words into short sentences.

He became calmer and more content. His nighttime tranquilizer allowed him to sleep nine to twelve hours through, and he still took one daytime nap (one to one-and-a-half hours).

During Brad's first eighteen months our family has had a great deal of adjusting to do. Things have not been pleasant. As parents we want happiness, good times, and a really nice family life for our children. It has been difficult and sometimes impossible to do things as a family. Even a picnic or a short trip to the zoo can turn into complete chaos.

Luckily for us, our children's problems have been diagnosed early. While things are just beginning with Brad, Diane has made tremendous strides during the past six months. Her new medication and her special school — plus maturity — have made her a new little girl. There is no denying that she still has problems. But we, as a family, are learning to handle them.

As parents of these two children, we accept their disabilities and are working to help the children adjust. While we have bad times, we do try to handle them.

The greater family adjustment problem seems, rather, to

be with the grandparents. We hear everything from "poor little dears" to "you're being too lenient," "you're spoiling them," "a little discipline would straighten them out." But we have been both routes. We do not feel sorry for the "poor babies," and we know that more punishment will not keep them from doing many of the things they do. We handled the grandparents as nicely as possible. For one set we would usually acknowledge that there is a problem and let them be sympathetic. For the other set of grandparents we would just ignore their comments completely, letting the words go in one ear and out the other. Of course, we voiced our frustrations to one another later, but in their presence it just seems best to keep quiet.

It has also been difficult to explain our problems to friends. If we try to describe what Diane does we hear, "But, all children do that." It is difficult to explain that it is not just what Diane does, but the amount of it that is the problem. Our pediatrician explained that it is a matter of degree. We handled these problems with friends in much the same way as we did with the grandparents — let it go in one ear and out the other (at least in their presence.)

Finally we adjusted to the fact that both family and friends, not living with hyperactivity, could not possibly understand the strain under which we were living. We made another adjustment: we decided to follow the counsel of our pediatrician and other experts in the field and to ignore criticisms of both family and friends.

So, what are we doing now? How do we handle the present?

First of all, we know what our problems are — we have a diagnosis. In four and one-half years we have been through many horrible days with Diane, through many days we throught literally would never end. And we have *many* pleasant memories, too. Now, with her, we can see the dawning of much better times.

This past year we have grown, as a family, in understanding. We know that we must help Diane to help herself. She must be helped to modify her behavior and to channel her energy into useful, meaningful activity.

At present, she attends school each weekday morning. The

environment there is quite structured, and there is much individual instruction. In fact, Diane's entire program is individualized for her, to help her with the specific disabilities she has.

During her school hours, Brad gets more individual attention at home. His fine motor skills were almost nil a few months ago. Now (age twenty months), he is beginning to make towers of six blocks, and he can stack rings in order on a stick. Still, he cannot really sit still for a story; but we are working on it. He at least does enjoy looking at books now. This extra time alone with Mama is definitely helping him.

After school, when lunch is over, Brad takes a short nap (forty-five minutes), and Diane has a quiet time — reading, coloring, painting, working on various skills, or just playing quietly. This is her time alone with Mama.

Things are more hectic after Brad's nap, for we never know how he will be. Some days he is a real bear — irritable and impossible to deal with. Other days he will play and be fairly calm.

Of course, Diane has plenty of bad afternoons, too. We sway with the punches. Things are great if both children have a good day; but if both have a bad day, Mama really has her work cut out. Normal squabbles between siblings become, in this household, magnified and continuous.

If things are going well, Diane has reached a point now (age four-and-a-half years) that she may visit with a friend or have a friend over in the afternoon. These play sessions are very good for her, and she is beginning to develop some sense of independence; she will walk to a nearby friend's house and back home again without Mama. Brad's visits with friends more often occur during Diane's school hours, unless these are family visits where the mothers visit with each other while the children play. Such visits in the afternoon, of course, include Diane.

Regardless of how the day has gone earlier, by four or four-thirty, some medication has worn off and the children are becoming tired. Life becomes quite hectic! Both children get wild. Their activity level increases and is very hard to work around.

It is almost impossible to have a nice family evening meal,

so things work out better if the children eat earlier than we do. Week nights we generally eat after they are in bed, while we attempt a family supper on Saturdays and Sundays.

After dinner comes one of the greatest benefits of Diane's new medication program and routine. Bedtime is seldom a hassle; she goes to bed most nights between 7:30 and 8:00 P.M. with no argument. Brad's bedtime is the same as Diane's. While it takes lots of energy to get Brad dressed for bed, he does not fight going to bed as Diane did for so long. Perhaps it is the tranquilizer, or perhaps it is a strictly followed routine that helps us with this bedtime procedure.

We have found that adhering to a fairly rigid regime really helps with our children. They know what to expect, and hence they behave better. We definitely have more problems with them on days when we relax our routine or do something special or different.

Much of what works for us now was found by trial and error. We certainly are trying not to repeat with Brad mistakes we made in handling Diane's problem. Hopefully we will see greater self-control in him younger than we saw it in Diane. At any rate, we have learned some things to do and many things not to do. For example, we do not give in to Brad's tantrums just to shut him up. We don't spank him as much as we did Diane, but we try to be firm. Often she did not know why she was being spanked. We spank Brad, but only when he knows why. In spite of possible side effects we placed Brad on medication at a much younger age. We overprotected Diane. Now we try to expose both children to more social situations, but attempt to limit overstimulation, which may occur in restaurants and crowds.

We try, as adults, to get away more in the evening. The children do very well for a good sitter because they have undivided attention (she does not have housework to do, too). The break is good for all of us.

Another thing that helps is to have the children play outdoors as much as possible. Fresh air and outdoor activity are beneficial both from a health standpoint and for the calming effect some activities have on them. Sandbox and water play are especially good "calmers." The more vigorous outdoor play—swinging, riding tricycles, running, pulling wagons, and so on—helps them work off excess energy. A good variety of activity toys, both indoors and out, is both useful and necessary with our children. These include spring horses, hoppity horses, bouncing rubber balls, horses with wheels, little riding vans, and pull toys. Many of these serve a dual purpose, as they are good for developing fine or gross motor control.

Indoors, a chalk board or easel and plenty of paper provide excellent opportunity for development; and they provide a calming down time. Books and other quiet-time supplies are also essential.

In addition to times of high activity followed by quiet-down times, our children need help in developing proper social skills. Diane has both school and play times with friends. Brad has begun to benefit from activities at the church nursery. One day each week he stays there while Mama enjoys "Mother's morning out." He also stays in the nursery during church on Sunday. Diane was unable, at Brad's age, to handle the stimulation of a large group of children, and we could not leave her in the nursery. Now, during this past six months, she has become able to handle Sunday School. In fact, she loves it and does not want to miss.

Diane's social skills have improved along with her ability to handle stimulation. At present we are hopeful that Diane will be able to enter a regular (but well-structured) nursery school next fall. Her teachers are well pleased with her improvement (as are we) and have recommended this move. They feel it will help her grow and be better prepared (hopefully) for public school. Her continued mornings away should allow me to give Brad some of the extra attention he needs, too.

These children do need lots of extra attention. While we do give them as much of our time as possible, and while things are much better now than they were six months ago, it will be a long fight. Both children are very easily overstimulated. When this happens, it is *very* difficult to calm them down. It is especially difficult when one of them comes in particularly overstimulated and, in turn, overstimulates the other. No amount of routine completely overcomes this stimulation problem.

Overstimulation especially occurs when we try to do special things as a family. Any break in routine—a trip to the zoo, a picnic, a home project, a particularly busy Mama (or Daddy)—can, and often does, send the children soaring.

We try to plan special activities and hope for the best. Many times we are happily surprised and things go quite well. We are really pleased when things do go well, for all children need fun times in order to be happy, well-adjusted little people.

How lucky we are! Our little people are bright and affectionate. We attempt to return their affection in *big* doses. For, as with all learning disabled children, ours must have that most of all—*love.*

In advising other parents of learning disabled children, no matter how slight or how great the disability, we would say:

> Know as much as possible about their problems;
>
> Seek professional and expert lay help (help for your child and help for you, for you must learn to cope with the problems you face with your child);
>
> Give your child *understanding;*
>
> Give hime *time;*
>
> Know when to hold on and when to let go (for these children must have a chance to develop and to "fly from the nest");
>
> And, most of all, give your child *love.*

In conclusion, I want to point out what helped me most to cope with the problems of having *two* hyperactive children. It was my husband. Although he became aware that there was a problem a bit later than I did, as soon as he was aware he was right there. Some parents have lots of marital troubles over having hyperactive children, but we had none between us. He started observing the children, he gave his support and understanding. He was as much involved in coping with the problems as I was. There were other things I did to cope, such as cry, talk too much about the problem with friends, read incessantly about the problem, and counsel with the director of

Diane's school, but my husband was and is my major source of strength.

MATTHEW

This is the story of an adopted child, now seven. Hyperactivity and other forms of learning disabilities occur more frequently in adopted children and this is one of the reasons it is important to tell Matthew's story. It is quite possible this situation occurs more with adopted children because of the potential lack of consistent pre-natal care on the part of people who expect to give up their infants. Matthew's mother also emphasizes the necessity of an understanding pediatrician and the special needs schools that are now developing. Matthew has come a long way and they have come a long way themselves, so much so they feel that if they would ever consider adopting another child, they would ask for a hyperactive child.

Though I am happily married, I am writing this from a mother's point of view...no, from *my* point of view, of *my* situation. I am sure if my husband were writing this story, though we have shared many of the incidents, feelings, and so on, it would be told in an entirely different light.

I am the mother of a hyperactive child. As a mother I am not always the picture of patience, and being harassed at times by an unrelenting, compulsively active child does not bring out the best in me. In addition, I have lived with all the guilt and resentments that this condition can cause. However, two things in my favor are a strong faith in God and a good sense of humor...I need them both.

To go back a bit:

We were so excited! The adoption agency had called on a Friday to say that our boy had arrived, was six weeks old, and was doing well. We could come down on Tuesday morning to see him and meet with the case worker. We then were to spend some time (overnight, to be exact) discussing the child and what we had learned about him and his biological parents. If we decided that this was indeed "our boy," then we could come Wednesday morning, with clothing and wraps, and our family would then number three.

Wayne and I were in our early thirties and had been married for four years. We were very elated that our first (and as it turned out, our only) child was about to enrich our lives. We arrived at the adoption home, eager indeed to see our prospective son. We were taken to the nursery window and the nurse held him up for us to see. Even at one day less than six weeks, his arms, legs, and head were all in motion. An omen of what was to come, if ever there was one! He seemed determined to give us his best performance, and we were impressed. He seemed as eager to be with us (or so we interpreted) as we were to have him with us. We talked with our case worker and the director of nurses at the agency and were given all available information, except the names of the parents. Knowing that the agency would either release the child that day or provide living quarters for my husband (who wasn't about to leave without that boy!), we had come prepared with bag and baggage for our Matthew. They understood, and he did come home with us.

He was a beautiful child to look at, a delight to behold. He had the normal cranky time in the evenings, and for about two weeks he required a feeding in the wee hours of the morning. This was just long enough to give us the memory of the experience without its becoming a chore.

In the early months Matthew was absolutely no problem at all. He slept well; he ate well; he was a happy, gurgling child. He turned over by himself by two-and-a-half months of age, cut four teeth by the time he was four months old, sat up alone at about six months. Everything seemed perfectly normal. I remember checking a copy of Dr. T. Berry Brazelton's book, *The First Twelve Months,* and finding that Matthew was in some activities in the slow category, in others in the normal category, and in still others in the advanced categories. Very balanced, I thought.

The only growth process that struck us as different was the development of his modes of mobility. He developed what we called his fish-flop traveling system. With head and chest just off the floor, he supported himself by his hands and arms. He would bend his left leg as close as possible to his body, dig in with his toes, and give a mighty push. He could move as fast as lightning that way, and did for a couple of months. Then one day in his seventh month, he crawled—and never again were we to see the fish-flop. All of this struck us as perfectly normal, especially since we had no other child in our family with whom to compare him. Matthew's pediatrician took his constant movement in the office and during examination as something that you deal with—nothing to be alarmed about. As Matthew grew, however, there was more and more to be "dealt with." The good books on child rearing tell you that when a child returns again and again to the same undesirable activity, such as shredding magazines or papers, you are to redirect his attention or remove this from the location—or remove the possibility of the undesirable activity, that is, remove the magazines and papers. Since we did not believe in removing everything that caught Matthew's attention, I did an awful lot of "redirecting" and "relocating" of Matthew. I did finally resort to spanking hands and spanking bottom. Since Matthew was also blessed with a very high tolerance of pain, physical punishment didn't work so well either. How many tears of frustration I shed!

Matthew continued to sleep well and eat well and cut teeth with no problem, but he was constantly in motion. Even by the age of two years, when I thought he should be enthralled with "Sesame Street" on television, he would condescend to watch for about two or three minutes at best. Nothing kept his attention. I would try to read to him, share picture books with him, teach him the names of objects—all to no avail. He wasn't interested for more than a split second, it seemed. Matthew would painstakingly take almost every toy apart, investigate anything that was in his reach and some things that were not, and step on anything that was in his way. We have some friends who nicknamed him "Tank" because he just rolled over any obstacle that stood between him and his desired destination. He was not malicious in his actions; he was simply single-minded. All of my well-intending friends and relatives would say, "If you'd just show him who's boss," or "He's just a boy!"

Matthew did have one development problem that gave me no end of concern, and that was his lack of language. He said *Mommy, Daddy, dog, bye-bye*—and that was about it. He seemed unable or uninterested in developing any more vocabulary. He just didn't talk. When he was two-and-a-half years of age I asked the doctor about this and was told that if he did not begin to talk by the time he was three years of age, then examinations and tests would be made to determine the reason, but that I was not to worry about it until that time. Believe it or not, about three months later, Matthew began to talk. He did not form his words well and still has some special language problems. He did cut his double-syllable words in half many times - for example, *curt* for *curtain, Jees* for *Jesus.*

He also went through a biting period that almost drove me up the wall. I could understand it when he was frustrated and up against greater size or demands than he could handle, but I could not understand it when in a nursery situation at church he went over to a little girl who had not annoyed him or challenged him in any way and bit her so hard that it broke the skin. I now understand that it was not the little girl who was overwhelming him, but the situation: too much noise, too much activity, too much color, too many children, and too little structure or guidance. All of these things were hitting his senses all at once with equal impact. He could not handle it and struck out at the first thing he saw. I'm sure he too was bewildered by his actions and had no way of understanding or explaining himself. Another time, a child who was larger than he put a demand on him in a play situation that he could not handle. Because he was unable verbally to express himself (his feelings or position), he bit the boy out of frustration and the inability to communicate.

All of these things happen, I am sure, in the lives of most children Matthew's age. The individual incidents were not so alarming as the degree of frequency and consistency with which they happened. I suspected hyperactivity but had no medical opinion to support my feelings. I was told "he's just alert and inquisitive," and a book on child management was recommended to me. I was convinced that it was more than alertness and inquisitiveness (both of which are two of his finer characteristics) that would cause a child to run in the house or dance in circles until perspiration poured off his face because he *had* to use some of the energy that was building up inside him. This occurred most often in days when he had to be inside because of bad weather. It seemed that he absolutely had to have some kind of play involving running, jumping, hopping, or other such large motor skills.

All of this time he also was having to deal with our demands on him, which sometimes were beyond his capabilities. About the time I became convinced that our boy was truly hyperactive we moved to the Indianapolis area and I finally, with God's help I am convinced, came in contact with an excellent pediatrician who understood my child's condition. May God grant him a long, fruitful life for his interest and efforts in behalf of a large number of children who would otherwise be tagged as rebellious, obstinate, undisciplined, ornery, disagreeable and, in general, unwanted. And certainly unappreciated. After the time I was ready to throw in the towel, I made an appointment with Matthew's pediatrician for a consultation. I had been taking Matthew to him for only about seven or eight months, and he had never mentioned hyperactivity to me. But when I came in for a consultation with him, not an appointment for Matthew, he simply came into the room with a form in his hand and asked me to complete it before we began talking. I did, and during the consultation it came to light that he was certain that Matthew was hyperactive but had not mentioned the possibility, waiting for me to initiate the subject. It seems that many parents do not want their child labeled hyperactive or hyperkinetic and do not want him medicated in any way. I simply wanted help for a little boy who had a lot going for him, but needed help in some areas. When it had been determined earlier in his life that his legs and feet needed extra support, we did not hesitate to put him in braces for a year, and when it was determined that he needed some teeth pulled, we didn't hesitate to take him to a pedodontist. If special education and medication were what it took to help him develop to his potential, we certainly would not deny him that either.

The good doctor suggested that I talk to the director of a special school for learning disabled children. I did and in a very short time Matthew was enrolled and attending three hours a day three times a week. Matthew's class was composed of six hyperactive boys taught by a super, very patient and loving teacher and an aide.

One of the first requirements for the school was a diagnostic evaluation by the psychologist who worked with the children. On the Stanford Binet Intelligence Scale, Matthew obtained a mental age of three years two months, one full year behind his chronological age. His IQ was 73, which indicated functioning within the borderline range—borderline range between minimally retarded and slow learner. This did not represent Matthew's intellectual potential, but it did reflect his level of functioning. He was highly distractible, very hyperactive, and openly negative during the testing, climbing on tables and throwing objects to try to elude testing. Matthew's gross motor skills (balancing, hopping, running) and fine motor skills (scissoring, drawing, writing, stacking blocks) were impulsive and uncontrolled. Although he was able to string beads and build with blocks at the three-year level and to sort objects at the three-and-a-half level, he was unable to copy either a line or a circle at the three-year level. His avoidance of paper/pencil tasks would make it very difficult to develop increased control in that area. Due to his strong rejection of all tasks involving pictures or books, the psychologist was able to obtain only a partial evaluation of Matthew's language and comprehension abilities, but she estimated them to fall within the three-to-three-and-a-half year level. Matthew's best performances were obtained on visual matching of identical objects and visual memory of objects from previous tasks (four-year level), which did not involve verbal directions or require verbal responses.

During the first term at the special school, Matthew physically attacked other children and the teacher by biting, hitting, or throwing objects. He simply was unable to control his impulses, handle any demands that would stretch his abilities, or cooperate for any length of time with his peer group. It was not a pleasant time for his teachers or for us. Matthew was not at this time on any medication. The director of the school wanted to see Matthew in his natural state in order to compare what benefits accrued from a structured environment in class. Then, if medication were required, a comparison would be available as to the changes brought about by structured environment plus the medication. When it was determined that the structured environment, even in a small group and with very capable teachers and aides, was not going to make any measurable difference, medication was prescribed in the form of Ritalin. When the proper dosage was determined, the Ritalin worked beautifully. It allowed him to show alertness and spontaneity, and at the same time it helped him sort out some of the impulses that were being simultaneously received by his brain. He was still highly distractible, but with redirection and improved concentration he began to progress.

In very few children, I am told, is the reaction so favorable to the first medication tried. Either we were extremely lucky, our doctor extremely good in his selection of medication and dosage, or God knew we were hanging on to the last knot in the rope and needed assistance quickly. You may choose any or all of the above.

A follow-up evaluation some three months later showed marked improvement in his behavior. Whereas during the first evaluation Matthew had presented problems of speech delay, low frustration tolerance, short attention span, and provocative and acutely hyperactive behavior outbursts, the psychologist had this to say about Matthew's second visit to her office:

> Although Matthew initially clung to his mother when he entered the clinic, he did not resist being cuddled and carried to my office and willingly sat down upon request. In contrast to his previous hyperactivity, he was quite attentive and cooperative. Resistance was minimal and occurred only on paper/pencil and abstract expressive language tasks, items which were quite difficult for him. However,

> perseveration was much more apparent and he became distractible when presented with multiple visual stimuli.
>
> On the Stanford Binet Intelligence Scale, Matthew obtained a mental age of three years six months, which was optimized to a mental age of three years ten months through demonstrations, redirection and extension of time limits. A significantly lower score was obtained on the Peabody Picture Vocabulary Test, due to his inability to inhibit responses to all pictures presented. While the obtained test scores are not considered to be reliable predictions of future potential, they do reflect a continuing delay of one-half to one year in conceptual development in spite of the behavioral improvements obtained with medication.

Matthew's third evaluation came a little over a year later and indicated that he continued to show significant developmental delays in spite of his marked behavioral improvements with medication. His test results, as on all previous testings, were very scattered. In this case his abilities and knowledge ranged from a four-year level to almost six-year level. His best performances were on tasks involving fine motor movements, copying models, and pointing responses, with much lower scores on items requiring receptive and expressive language skills, arithmetic concepts, and drawing. In contrast to his previous impulsive and negative behavior during testing, this time he was very quiet and noticeably anxious on verbal tasks, often covering his mouth and usually speaking in whispers. He worked steadily on performance tasks, but his manual dexterity was poor, with clumsy handling of materials in spite of purposeful movements. His classroom reports at that time indicated that Matthew was continuing to show improvement in social behavior and willingness to participate in classroom routines. He particularly enjoyed gross-motor games (kickball, climbing, and running activities) and working with small play tiles and was more willing to attempt paper/pencil tasks. Impulsive and aggressive behavior occurred infrequently and usually followed provocation, but his progress in language development continued to be extremely slow.

So far in Matthew's story, Matthew has been the primary

focal point. Now let's shift the spotlight to two other people who were directly involved in all of this—Wayne and me. What had this done to our relationship? What conflicts had this brought about? How did we handle them? The answers to these questions are: Sometimes helped, sometimes hindered; lots; sometimes poorly, sometimes magnificently. For a bit more detail in these areas let me tell you something of our makeup. As previously stated, Wayne and I were about thirty when we adopted Matthew. We were very, very happy to finally find "our" boy, but he did bring about considerable changes in our life-style. For one thing Wayne and I had held responsible jobs. We enjoyed our careers and each respected the other's. We are home-loving people; we enjoyed having dinner in or out with friends, playing bridge or golf, having evenings to ourselves in our home, and being very involved in church activities. One would think that a baby would bring no real necessary adjustment to this scene. Wrong. Someone else now decided schedules and presented a different priority. Matthew. His behavior and development were not exactly as we had thought they would be—and each of our reactions was not as the other one had thought it should be.

Our conflicts did not come during Matthew's infancy. He was a sweet, beautiful baby and we adored him. The inconveniences we experienced were absolutely nothing compared to the utter joy we felt in having him. I thought nothing of providing 90 percent of the care required by Matthew, because I was with him all the time. Wayne, like most fathers, saw him only at night and on weekends. Wayne also traveled some, and that cut down on his availability. He did, however, awaken much more quickly in the night than I, because he is a much lighter sleeper. Sometimes he would hear Matthew, take care of his needs, and come back to bed, and I would never be the wiser.

Actually our conflicts came when Matthew became a toddler. Part of the problem was Matthew's development and behavior, but a great deal of it has to be placed squarely at our feet. We simply had standards previously arrived at and it was very difficult for us to adjust. This included standards for Matthew and for each other. For instance, when Matthew was about two years old there arose a conflict between us as to the time Wayne would spend with Matthew. From both points of view it looked like this:

WAYNE:	I hold a very responsible, sometimes very demanding job, and I need my Saturdays to play golf with the fellows. The golf usually lasts until around 1:30 P.M.; I come home, rest awhile, then go out and mow the lawn. I come in, take a shower, dress and am ready for dinner and relaxation for the rest of the evening. The following day is taken up with church activities both in the morning and evening, with a nap on Sunday afternoon while the baby is asleep. What more can I do? I work to provide a living for my family, I mow the lawn, and I participate and, at times, lead in the spiritual activities and growth of my family.
MY VIEWPOINT:	You are gone each day and some nights, and the other nights you come home and dwell on what has happened in your life during the day. On Saturday you are either on the golf course, furiously mowing the lawn, or asleep. Sundays are well taken up with church activities. Where is the time for family life? Where is any uninterrupted time with your boy and your wife? Don't you realize what you are missing? And, quite truthfully, where is any time for me to do something by myself? You direct your time totally; I direct none of mine.

I came to the very painful decision in my own mind that what was really wrong was that Wayne wanted to *have a son* but he did not want to *be a father*. I could not reconcile that.

Also, both of us expected more of Matthew than he could produce, both behaviorally and intellectually. We were at times impatient with his lack of "potty training," his lack of communication, and his persistence in nonappropriate activities. These activities could be anything from tearing a book he was enjoying (due to either carelessness or impulsive muscle reaction) to resorting to unacceptable behavior in order to get attention, even if it was negative attention. He was immature for his age level; that is, more like a two-year level at four years of age. At other times none of this bothered us. I am sure our lack of consistency did not help Matthew. I also thought Wayne expected much too much in the way of instant obedience from Matthew. After all, the child was only two, three, or four years old. He wasn't an adult. I thought he was too tough on Matthew. One of the main problems was that Wayne was always more *affectionate* than he was *effective.* He had only two ways of communicating with, or being a father to, Matthew—either to cuddle him or to be harsh with him. There was no level ground for Matthew—no consistency on which he could depend. Either his father was being lovey-dovey to him or was rejecting him by his harshness. It was very hard for Matthew to guess which way his father would be at a given time, and I have often seen him guess wrong and suffer the consequences.

Wayne had been a middle child. In his adult life he was never around children more than for a short visit. He really knew almost nothing about children and their development and thought it was ridiculous that a person could learn anything about fatherhood from a book. I, on the other hand, had good rapport with children, having been around them all my life—in the family, babysitting, and teaching Bible classes and just enjoyed them immensely. However, I was impatient at times and was becoming more resentful all the time that Wayne was not pulling his share. This also led, at times, to my thinking of Matthew as an intrusion into my life.

Another stress factor was provided by the fact that Wayne and I were above average in intelligence and in our language abilities. This made Matthew's developmental delay and lack of language harder to accept. We had great expectations for our son. We had expected that he would be born with all the abilities and potentials of a child of at least slightly higher than average IQ and physical capabilities. The parents of a brain-damaged child often find it difficult to drop down to the communication, comprehension, and activity level of their offspring. This increases the stress level on both the child and the marriage. Add to this that hyperactive children do not simply see an activity and then do it like other children do. Because of lack of muscular and impulse coordination, hyperactive children have to be taught how to do a lot of things that other children simply do naturally, like swinging, hopping, riding a tricycle, or holding a crayon or a fork. This is yet another stress factor on the child and the marriage.

This is not to say that ours was an unhappy house. It wasn't. But when it was unhappy, these are the things that made it so. At times there was tension, sometimes high tension. But it came quickly and left quickly. We were outspoken with each other, but it was practically to no avail—as neither of us changed perceptibly.

Matthew was four years old when he was diagnosed psychologically as falling in the borderline slow-learner range. His difficulties had caused terrific strains within the family. My husband and I have gone through many anxious moments because of the strain on each of the relationships represented within our family. I am sure that separation or divorce would have been more strongly considered if the Bible and our religious brotherhood did not teach this as out of reach. It simply wasn't an option available to us. And also there was our own hardheadedness about coping and conquering, but most of all there is the deep love that flows among all three of us for each other. But believe me, though I am not proud of it and though God's Word teaches against separation, divorce, and child abuse, I have been sorely tempted by all three in my weaker moments.

Matthew is now six years of age. He is still in the special school, doing a classroom program within the prekindergarten-to-beginning level, with emphasis on basic preacademic concepts as well as formal academic training. A speech therapist works with the children once a week. His pediatrician keeps in close contact with the school director and psychologist. He is receiving the very best of care and education, we believe. He continues to need large amounts of praise and encouragement at home — and receives it. Loud noise levels, a lot of activity, and groups still tend to overwhelm him, but he is enjoying improvement in all areas. His verbalization is increasing rapidly (in other words, he chatters like a magpie!). His concepts are broadening and his language comprehension is improving. He delights in toys that require very fine finger manipulation and enjoys books tremendously.

Parents of minimally brain-damaged children do not enjoy triumphs of their children as frequently as parents of normal children. I personally think this makes our victories much sweeter, simply because they are harder to achieve and come less frequently.

Matthew is a very attractive, happy, alert, active, well-mannered six-year-old, secure in his knowledge that his parents love him very much. He is a very loving and giving child, and he does not have a malicious bone in his body. This, plus his lack of confidence in himself, makes him very vulnerable to hurt and rejection by other children and adults alike. His outward appearance belies his inward condition. In fact, many of our friends do not see any indication of his hyperactivity. He loves his school — all of it: the teachers, the activities, being with the class members. He loves his home, his parents, his relatives, his toys, his dog. He can be as active as a grasshopper, but he can also sit and play for long periods of time with his toys, his record player and records, his books. He travels beautifully and is never bored or fidgety in the car. He becomes very excited about new adventures such as a ferry boat ride, eating at a new restaurant, or a roller-coaster ride with his dad at a Disneyland-type setting.

Wayne is fast becoming my candidate for Father of the Year. For the past year or so he has developed a very fine relationship with our son. They spend a great deal of time together and enjoy many activities together, as we do as a family. When time and job responsibilities allow, Wayne even car pools the four children in our area and enjoys them all tremendously. Recently Wayne even took Matthew on an all-day, out-of-town trip to King's Island, the Disneyland-type setting I referred to previously. The two of them had a great time, all by themselves. Two years ago this would not have even been considered, much less undertaken.

I do not profess to know all the reasons for this but can only guess a few: Wayne has grown a great deal as a person and as a father; he has learned to appreciate what Matthew is and to enjoy tremendously his successes. Neither of us is nearly as concerned as before that our parental image with others might suffer because of Matthew's disability. On the other hand, Matthew has become more of a communicative person, with a progressive understanding of the world about him, including his dad. They are able to enjoy more things together as Matthew grows a little older. His improved coordination permits them to enjoy more games and physical activities; his increased vocabulary allows more expression of thoughts, ideas, and impressions; Matthew is more a "person" than he is a "baby."

We have learned to improve the atmosphere in our home by realizing that there are times when one parent or the other needs to leave the situation and "relocate" to another area. For instance, mornings seem to be a difficult time for Matthew. Though he gets up in the mornings with a great big smile on his face and happily comes hopping down the hall to the breakfast area, you can almost bet your last dollar that within three minutes something will occur that will bring on either whining or crying from Matthew. This drives Wayne up the wall. Even though it may last for only a minute or two (and sometimes it goes much longer), he finds it very hard to handle. The only two acceptable alternatives are: learn to handle it correctly or remove yourself from the situation. We tried switching off when or before this occured and it worked quite well.

I might add that Matthew can manipulate quite well, and once he picks up on an arrangement like this he can work one parent against the other if it is to his advantage. We put a stop to this manipulation by taking turns at being in charge and car pooling. Every other week I take the morning responsibilities: I prepare, serve, and clean up after the breakfast; I prepare the lunches; I see that Matthew does the necessary ablutions; I lay out his clothes for him, if he doesn't choose them himself; and I am responsible for keeping both of us on schedule. Matthew has caught on now that he has no higher court of appeals and there is no change of venue—the parent who starts with him when he wakes up is in charge of him until he gets to school. This doesn't allow much maneuvering room.

This does not mean that there is always a problem situation in our home. Not by any means. Many days are as normal as those of any other parent. It is just that when times are not normal we have learned to use slightly different methods than other parents—and we have to use them more often.

However, with all the stress, extra expense, and extra effort necessary to maximize Matthew's abilities and knowledge, he is the light of our lives. We love and enjoy him tremendously, and he has taught us to appreciate and delight in happenings that would have otherwise eluded us. In other words, he brings joy to our lives. We hope we are becoming the parents that Matthew deserves and that each of us can enjoy and respect. We hope we can provide him the environment and motivation he needs to reach his full potential.

Together we have learned that everyone has a handicap. Maybe it is physical, mental, emotional, or is in personality or appearance. Some are more easily diagnosed and treated than others. All of us are working on ours.

PETER

Peter's mother wrote this story about her ten year old son on her own since she is now separated from her husband. In probably no other story in this book is the terrible "aloneness" so evident as is expressed in the thoughts that we see go through her mind. Not only did she have to face the daily problems with Peter, but those of the family too. Peter's hyperactivity did make a major contribution to the eventual separation, but it also contributed to his mother's acceptance of the family problem and finally the development of necessary daily strategies that make their life today so much more pleasant. A compounding problem that is emphasized more in the story than any of the others is the tragically cruel attitudes of "friends" who are often inconsiderate enough to set up their own "normal" children as the accepted norm. Perhaps this story is as much about Peter's mother as it is about him, for she is creating a successful person out of him by elevating herself. Peter has a five year old brother.

This child has the same feelings as all of us, but we cannot respond to him with the usual behavior.

After five years of marriage, it seemed having a baby might make things better. Besides, everyone else seemed to be doing it, and I might even like it. I didn't realize until later that

I wasn't a 'born mother.' Conceiving the baby was easy, but the pregnancy was long. The fetus was active with sporadic and jerky movements. Since I was still working in Boston, we would drive daily into the city. Jeff, my husband, had just purchased a diesel Land Rover which is built for the African terrain. It had tight springs and the diesel engine created a deafening roar. It was the combination of these two things that caused the fetus to move with frantic activity for an hour after each ride. It did not surprise me to read later that unborn children do hear sounds and such a loud noise would have certainly been uncomfortable to his ears.

Peter's birth was induced with medications, which also put me to sleep for the six hours of labor, so it was suggested that my husband go home to wait for the new child's arrival. In the brief period before I fell asleep, the feeling of being alone, frightened and not in control of my own body was to mark my memory. When I awoke, it was as if nothing had happened. The male child I saw gave me no feelings of fulfillment nor did it express a kind of love bound between a man and myself. I felt guilty for my lack of enthusiasm for this child and the event of a birth; an indefinable sadness seemed to surround me. To help alleviate these feelings, I did nurse Peter in hopes of giving him closeness and nurturing.

Coming home brought the usual onlookers, gifts and comments, but not the usual "Isn't he cute." Peter wasn't cute like the babies you see on television, nor did he have the blond hair and blue eyes that I expected. His hair was already dark brown as were his eyes. Peter looked exactly like his father and I really wondered why I deserved that after carrying him for those nine long months. It was devastating to hear from everyone, "He certainly doesn't look like you." Peter cried a lot. He usually started about six o'clock just as I was trying to cook dinner. It didn't cease until he would finally sleep from exhaustion about 10 o'clock. The crying made the new father very nervous and it was as though Jeff expected me to make him stop. I did all I could but nothing would help. Pacifiers, warm water with Karo, or nursing gave no relief. Peter would refuse all but the nursing. I thought I had to endure all.

During the night it would all start again. Peter would awaken with a sudden shrill cry, as if he was in pain. I would try to nurse him as we rocked. I would hold him or put him on his stomach and rub his back. This helped momentarily but never for long. I could hear the sounds of distress coming from his body. If I tried to cuddle Peter, he would arch his back and push himself backwards. He seemed to reject all that I could think of. When he did fall asleep, he would sometimes awaken just as I lay him down, or the creaking noise of the floor would startle his oversensitive ears. I didn't have a full night's sleep that whole year.

The constant night crying did not endear this strange creature to Jeff who was an acheiving, upcoming, hardworking man. I felt a great sadness with the lack of Peter's father holding him or touching him. I know it isn't easy for a man to hold or diaper a child, but I wished once Jeff would have said he wanted to learn. I felt forced to protect and love Peter. But Peter met neither Jeff's or my criteria of what our child was supposed to be. I wasn't sure Jeff had even wanted to be a father. When Peter was just home from the hospital, Jeff had said, "It will take twenty years before Peter is grown and we are alone again." There was no joy and excitement over his son.

Since I could not satisfy Peter's crying and fussing, friends and relatives were quick to assume it was because I wasn't able to supply enough milk. I became so nervous that first month that I borrowed a scale and found Peter was gaining weight at a good rate. This should have given me confidence that at least it was not me. But, my lack of confidence was to increase and the resentment toward this child to heighten with every unsuccessful attempt to satisfy his crying.

Peter had a distended stomach; everyone remarked on how bad it looked. He was a very colicky baby. The pediatrician had told me that the distention was due to weak stomach muscles. At four weeks, Peter was unable to have a bowel movement for a whole week. The pediatrician prescribed water and told me not to worry. I wished by the fourth night he could have been the one to stay up with the screams. Peter did have a bowel movement on the fifth evening and he couldn't have done anything that would have made me happier. He was not constipated as I would have expected. His stool was the same loose consistency that all nursing babies seem to have. Although this did not happen again, Peter was to have constipation problems during his first six years. Something had caused inability of his bowels to empty properly. Jeff and the pediatrician had made me feel it was my nervousness. I felt no one wanted to listen to me, and Peter was causing things to happen to me that were very unpleasant. There was no one for me to retaliate against. I had to suffer through each day and night, since I was the only one of Peter's parents who was responsible for the needs he *screamed* for. This infant sapped the very being from me!

I know that Jeff cared for Peter. It was just hard for me to feel this caring when every time Jeff was awakened in the night by Peter's cries, he would get so angry. "Why doesn't he sleep?" or, "I couldn't sleep at all last night and I have a very big day." "Every meal time it is guaranteed Peter will cry." Door-slamming or swearing were not uncommon. I would try to hustle this little fellow as far away as I could and almost pray for him to be quiet. Noises seemed to bother Jeff and his need for a tranquil home, I could not fulfill. Jeff's interest in sailing increased during this period. I was not surprised to hear him say, "It will be a long while before Peter can go with us." "Indeed," I thought to myself, "Jeff has not gained a son; he feels he has lost his wife!" I think he, too, resented Peter for intruding on his life.

At one point in the first three months, Peter's sleeping problem became too hard to cope with, so the doctor recommended phenobarbital. I recall the results were not instant sleep and my general hesitation in using medications resulted in a short trial. My dislike for medicines of this kind had absolutely no religious or moral grounds, but just a hesitation to put so much in a small child not knowing the results. My conscience constantly kept me from these medicines. They never solved *THE PROBLEM* — that *"this was not just an ordinary child."*

In the meantime, all my friends who had produced children at the same time had **'beautiful little geniuses'** who were adored and admired by all. These comments penetrated my heart since I felt I couldn't say this about Peter and, unfortunately, there were no adoring grandparents, relatives or father. He was seen as a collection of problems and no one wanted to love him for his sake, just because he was a new little human being.

Maybe, I began to feel the **total** responsibility to protect him from this critical world. He did develop, often normally: he smiled, rolled over at three months, crawled at six months and walked at one year. I'm sure he did this all on his own. In that first year I wondered about Peter a lot, but whenever it was suggested something was wrong I became defensive for both him and myself.

Even though Peter had a normal development physically, there were a few physical symptoms that indicated distress. His distended stomach with his colicky digestion was always apparent. When he learned to stand in his crib, he gnawed constantly at the wood. I could not guess whether this was due to nervous activity or frustration. He often banged his head against the end of the crib as he rocked back and forth on his hands and knees. Since Peter never sucked his thumb or took a pacifier, he had no way of relaxing.

During the second year, his sleeping habits and my doubts about my ability to take care of this child caused me to give him three different medications. All babies should normally be in bed asleep by at least seven or eight o'clock, but ten o'clock was unheard of. This was difficult for a tired father, not to mention a mother who was exhausted. Phenergan showed slight improvement. Dexedrine and Benzedrine showed nothing noticeable except some increase in activity. I now felt I was unable to do anything with Peter.

On one of our many trips to the pediatrician, I was told that Peter was hyperactive. His latent speech development, poor peer relations, poor family interaction, and high activity level fit into the pattern observed in hyperactive children. Peter's motor development was a problem and his reflexes were very active. He was a difficult and negative child who slept poorly, even to the point of often getting out of bed at night on his own. The doctor also saw Peter's bowel and bladder training as an important part of the overall problem. **How was I to cope with a hyperactive child?**

Only once during that second year did he speak a sentence. "I want to go outside." I could not believe he said this and he could not repeat it the next instant. At three years one month Peter visited his first psychologist. By then I felt especially incapable of handling this child. The psychologist described Peter as having poor speech, immature motor skills, and volatile nature that was easily triggered. The child was recommended for therapy and it was suggested he attend a Montessori School that would provide structure. The psychologist noted our marital problems and the fact that we, as two separate individuals, were so tied into our own problems that we were unable to give to this child. He recommended weekly counseling for us, but I was the only one who took the suggestion; my husband did not want to go. I saw a social worker for the remainder of that year, who seemed to hold me in equilibrium.

Peter's intellectual development appeared to be low normal to average with some indication there was a slow development due to an emotional block. I felt during this period that I was to blame and was the cause of all of our son's problems. Perhaps his inability to do things was because I was a poor teacher; I couldn't spank him, I couldn't love him, I felt maladjusted. I never completed anything; his negativism, tantrums, and distractibility caused me to join in his frenzy. I forgot what "normal" could be. I had to guess that some way, somehow things could be better. I would have liked someone, just one person, to understand me and tell me now and then I did something right. I wished for a little encouragement, but since there was no one I began to believe that my judgment had lost its worth.

Peter was now old enough for school, but cried and ran away from the car every time he was to go. He resisted in every way he could. Peter's report from the Montessori school showed only several satisfactory categories. He rated well in energy, along with his sense of rhythm and balance, and his muscular development. His articulation, acceptance of directions, participation, consideration, group interaction, individual work, listening, eye/hand coordination, orderly manner, concentration, attention to direction, and social adjustment all needed improvement. Can you imagine how I felt to see mostly "unsatisfactories" on his report?

On one occasion, Peter was not chosen to participate in a musical presentation that was to be videotaped. The teacher told me she felt he should not be included since his behavior was not reliable. It would be too difficult for him. I went home that day to one of my friends with sobs of anger, resentment and a deep hurt. The other children were all all right; they could go to Boston and do this thing for the T.V. My "friends" had bright kids, but why didn't I? I hated my "friends" and what their kids could do; of course, all this was inside me and I felt I must tell no one. I should not hate anyone. My father had told me that. Love everyone, he had told me. Maybe, that was why I felt I was a terrible failure as a mother, wife, and friend. I kept trying to love everyone and **I couldn't even love myself.**

Peter would not include me in any of his emotions, except anger. He had great difficulty in expressing himself. It was as if he wanted to say something but couldn't articulate his thoughts. I would try to guess what he wanted to say and fill in for him. That would often enrage him if I guessed the wrong thing. I never knew how he felt about things that happened to him. He could barely tell me when he didn't feel well. One day he was being taken care of by a "friend." I was going to my violin lesson. When I returned, I found he had ripped a good children's book apart. It appeared that he had been very angry at being left there, but it turned out he was sick and had felt poorly. The next week when I took him to the same "friend," he ripped another book apart. The "friend" was very unhappy, understandably, and she wanted me to replace the books. I had a hard time to feel anything but resentment for Peter. But, I got the message that he should not go to that house again. It became harder and harder to love Peter and he must have known how I felt. He told me when he was nine that I had never loved him. **He was right.**

My conscience was increasingly bothered by what was happening to this child. Why should a child scream when you send him off to school? Could this possibly be right? If you went out to dinner and the babysitter came, the child was horrified to see you leave to the point that he had to be restrained. Could this be security? It is hard to cope with and I can understand why my husband and others would say to leave him alone and he'd be all right when we left. It was true he *was* all right when I returned, but the knowledge that things could be better for the child haunted me daily. Meanwhile, close "friends" were sure he wasn't all right and needed medication. A relative felt I was too passive and needed to crack down on him. **In no way was I winning!**

Peter's school had a photography exhibit. All the children had been photographed by a woman as they were doing their work. Peter's two teachers were very anxious for me to see Peter's picture. He looked like he had a halo over his head. The remark, "That's one child who had no halo," was like a knife in my heart. These teachers will still remark: "We have never had a child like Peter."

The final report from the school verified Peter still had changeable emotional moods, social aggressiveness, an inability to relate to peers, an insistent *demand* for attention, and an obvious need for professional help. His reliance on adult assistance showed his lack of independence. It was emphasized during his second and third year of life that we indeed had a hyperactive child, a label I could not understand. Not one soul could tell me how to get out of this maze but just that I was in it.

> All things are now thought of in terms of—how can I suffer this, NOT how can the child suffer this confusion, rejection, resentment, and lack of ability and love.

In the summer of Peter's fourth year, the first major event was my brother's wedding. Peter was asked to be a ringbearer in the wedding, which was a boost to my ego though he did not know what it all meant. The reactions were predictable from all who knew him. My brother was the positive type and that helped me not give up. I borrowed a short suit and shirt and tie for Peter. We flew to Florida for the event and I expected whatever would be, would be. The woman in charge of the wedding took over for me, and to my uncontrollable sobs of joy Peter walked down that aisle alone. I had doubted his ability to do anything, but he had performed for someone else. He was unable to stand still for the whole ceremony, but I saw him for one moment as a cute little boy.

It was right after Peter's fourth birthday that the second

major event occurred. We moved to Connecticut. Peter seemed to have a new hope. He kissed his new house and said he loved it, a feeling he rarely ever experienced. I had left all the old "friends" with their bright kids. I had lots of time to think and to plan where I was. I decided to try out a few of the ideas I had observed my friends doing.

I tried coloring. He scribbled and avoided following suggestions. I began to reassess the pattern I had developed before our move of protecting the child from criticism by blaming myself or developing excuses. I had, during those first four years, tried to listen to what everyone's opinion was. I had read books and thus changed my mind daily or weekly whenever I saw any new hint of a solution. I lived in dread of each of Peter's tantrums. He did get his way often if he used this device on me.

I became pregnant that fall with courage that I would not have another child like Peter. The fetus acted less frantic and I believed this already indicated something was different. For this reason I seemed to care more for Peter that year. I wasn't trying to keep up with my old "friends," and I really wanted to believe Peter could be better. Some things I tried did improve. He became more able to build with legos, blocks, tinkertoys and sometimes surprised me with his results. His behavior still was not acceptable in his father's eyes. I began to prefer to give all my energy to Peter and spend little time with my husband. Peter, at least, needed me and I wanted to be needed by someone. Perhaps I did too much for Peter and this lead to criticism from Jeff.

Jeff worked day and night, was always tired, and the children's noise was too much for him. Jeff liked to putter around the house and fix things. So, on the weekends, Jeff had more projects than time. Our Saturday morning breakfasts were our conversation times, while the kids watched television. We would occasionally take a walk or ride together on Sunday. Those were the only times during the week that Jeff had with his family, including any special time with the boys. There might be a game of ball for 15 minutes or a little project with Peter, but I can't recall any longer periods of contact between Jeff and his father. After these special periods together, Jeff either felt the pressure of other projects or was tired. The times together were short and far between. Often on weekends Peter would do something that would cause Jeff to get very angry with him. Perhaps it was spilled milk, or something of Jeff's that was broken or misplaced. Peter might just be in Jeff's way trying to watch what he was doing. I felt sorry for Peter each time this happened, since often the anger was much greater than the deed. The idea I had developed in the last four years — that I did not want Peter to be influenced by Jeff — came constantly into my mind.

Peter was enrolled in nursery school that year. The teacher seemed very nice and I was able to talk about myself and my deficiencies in handling Peter. The teacher mentioned that Peter's lack of attention might be due to a hearing problem. So, off we went again and had not only psychological tests but two hearing tests. The psychologist with the public school system was so warm and kind that I felt she really liked Peter. She spoke of him as being a bright child in his responses to her directions and tests. That made me proud of him. He did have a hearing loss in one ear in the higher decibels.

When I was in my 8th month of pregnancy, Peter was playing outside one afternoon and came running in screaming. I thought at first he had hit his head, but he could not tell me what was hurt. My reactions at these times were always slow, ambivalent and certainly did not lead him to believe I cared. He continued to say he felt terrible and I waited, not quite believing he was hurt so much. He had some swelling in the shoulder area and could not be touched. The next day he could barely move, and was angry there was no one to help carry him to the car as I was eight months pregnant. I was supposed to bring Peter into the office and almost did but something made me insist that he be checked in the car. The Doctor said immediately there was a broken bone. He asked me to drive to the hospital where he could be put on a stretcher for Xray. Why had I not been able to hear my child say he was hurt and believe what he was trying to tell me? I felt real guilt that I couldn't even say to him, "I'm sorry I let you suffer so long." The collar bone had a complete fracture which kept Peter in bed for the week. Peter was a good patient, was quiet, and rested well. I told him many times I was sorry for what happened and tried to be loving and kind to him. Jeff cared too and wanted Peter to feel all right again.

During the year I was pregnant, I had enjoyed Peter. Our relationship was better than it had ever been. We had read books about babies and gone regularly to the library. I had continued to work with him on puzzles, books, building things and listening to records. It was just before the baby came I felt for the first time I wanted to run to Vermont to a little shack with the kids and leave Jeff, the big house, friends, family, money and just work at building a happy family.

When Eric was born, Peter was really proud. He loved his little brother and would tell everyone in the supermarket he had a new brother. That summer Jeff lost his job, my parents came to help me with the new baby and I really began to feel trapped and unsatisfied with my life and wondered if I could ever be able to relate to anyone correctly.

I began to think I wanted out of my marriage and pictured how things could be. I felt that my marriage would never improve and began to realize that my inability to follow through with Peter might be due to my struggle with Jeff. Jeff criticized everything I tried with Peter. I could do nothing right. This was love? He criticized my not following through on things, my disorganization at dinner time, and the way I handled the children. The more I was criticized the more I hurt, and lashed back at Jeff and sometimes even Peter. But I didn't want to hurt Peter; I wanted to help him. It was that summer I gave up on my marriage. In my heart it was gone. Peter needed help and I wanted to help him. I couldn't help Peter as long as I lived with Jeff. But I decided I would temporarily defuse myself and go on for another month.

> Peter was the reason I could not wait to change things at home. He would grow up in a home without love, with conflict and it would be too late for him to feel the other life if I waited much longer.

Peter entered kindergarten with his usual reluctance. He expected me to be nervous and I expected him to be reluctant. I followed my usual technique of telling the teacher all the problems so she wouldn't be surprised if he didn't perform. Peter had bowels which no longer emptied. The pediatrician put him on mineral oil, starting with 1 or 2 tablespoons. I was nervous about this as I had been brought up to worry about bowels, feet and teeth. I, of course, had to tell the teacher about this too. I just couldn't shut up.

His bowel problem ran its course of increased oil to the point of about 6 tbs. per day. I would often get up with Peter from the dinner table to go with him to the bathroom when he couldn't eat any more. I felt he could sit for a while on the toilet, and we would look at books or read. I tried to take off the pressure and hoped a routine pattern would be established. Jeff thought I was pushing him and resented my efforts. I did get results and he began to re-establish some peristaltic action in his intestines. The summer Peter was six, my mother was visiting and it was decided that we should make sure he was all right physically. Peter had a barium enema. I bought him a battery operated boat for $20 to get him to do this. He wanted to take it into the Xray room the next day. The doctor was cold and absolutely unresponsive and didn't act like he could have cared.

Peter wanted to show his new boat to the doctor, but that damn doctor ignored Peter. He was a busy person and had a schedule to meet. When Peter was frightened and didn't want to do the test, the doctor said he had never seen such a child. If Peter didn't do the test quickly, he would have to reschedule the test. I had already given Peter two prep enemas at home and I knew I didn't want to have the test rescheduled.

I wanted to run out of there. But I didn't leave. I watched them put that too large enema bulb into my terrified child. I had to tell Peter he had to do it. He did it for me. The test was negative. But my mother was satisfied even though I felt I had cursed my child once more.

> At first you feel as though anyone who is a doctor or teacher can tell you everything. The difficulty is to hold on to yourself and your intuitive instincts that are constantly being challenged by professionals.

I did have one person I could talk to in those days. She was my 82 year old violin teacher. She was a woman beyond description, sensitive to people, aware, modest, self-sufficient, artistic and understanding. When we would talk about Peter, she was a positive person who only believed in what could be done. She told me the stories about Einstein's problem and the fact he once was about to take a hammer to his little sister's head. Einstein's mother believed in him and took him out of school when all else failed. He talked late and is known to have had learning difficulties. She taught him herself and we know now he was a genius. My teacher's belief and encouragement gave me a positive feeling about myself. She meant a great deal to me. She also thought Peter was nice and he responded to her.

In first grade Peter seemed to do well enough, although the teacher was horrified one day when he exposed himself in their dismissal line. He still hated to go to school and I almost always had to drag him via car. The teacher was a vivacious type, structured and very friendly. She would try to tease him into getting his work done and she seemed to feel he was capable. He worked slowly and was distracted by any noise. He went weekly to have a period of social group play with the adjustment counselor. In January of that year, when Peter was seven, I called another professional, this time a pipe smoking, very expensive child psychiatrist. He recommended therapy and Jeff, Peter and I all went separately, and at unbelieveable costs. He prescribed Mellaril and later Benadryl for Peter, and again my own feelings made it difficult for me to give it to him. At one point, Peter refused to take the Mellaril and I thought perhaps he was feeling some reverse effects from the drug. He often complained of a stomach ache, and this time I listened to Peter and stopped the drug.

Peter refused to go to school at one point. I would dress him for school and he would undress as quickly as I got him dressed, then he would hide under the bed. I was torn between removing him entirely from school, or following the psychiatrist's advice of sending him regardless. At this stage, I felt desperately incapable of handling myself or the child. He did continue to go to school, although there were several days with hour long scenes at the classroom door. He first would balk at getting out of the car; I would get him to the classroom door; then, he wouldn't go in. The principal would tell me he was always fine once he was in school. There were also those looks that say—you know you're the cause of your child's problem and it's not the school.

Jeff had three job changes, two by necessity, during this four year period. The added psychological strain on Jeff and concerns for financial security may indeed have added a third dimension to Peter's already confused life. We returned to live near Boston the summer Peter was eight. I could see I had changed from being away from my old friends. I had been forced to think for myself and try to assume some of my own criteria for my life and goals for this child. I tried to be open to the world around me and stimulate some excitement for Peter. I bought French records and would play them as he woke up in the morning. Since they were for children he began to repeat the songs. I used other musical records, some with a spoken dialogue. Several he liked so well he would play them over and over. I tried to teach him his spelling words using any technique I could come up with. We even had a pillow fight one night as we spelled each word correctly. I wanted to keep him busy and take advantage of his energy. I think my husband saw me as a pusher and had his own historical reasons for disliking this pushiness. I would, as a result of my lack of commitment on this, be inconsistent. I was too changeable.

I had been happy in that house and school in Connecticut, as had Peter, and he hated leaving. Somehow we didn't see Peter's happiness in the same way he did. We were not slated to move into our house, which needed so much work, for several months but Peter was to attend a new strange school in that town. The events that followed were predictable. Peter felt alone, missed his former school, and began to have problems with his schoolwork. He was harder than ever to control. He demanded and became obsessed with lights and especially train crossing gate signals. I spent some time driving him to the train in time to see the crossing gates go down and up or he wasn't satisfied.

He threw things, destroyed many items, and took his problems out on his brother. The math homework that began to come home became more difficult to deal with. His recall of his basic math facts was inconsistent. I had a friend who had her child in a special school for learning disabled children and I was desperate to try and find another answer. When I first contacted this special school I was given many forms to fill out. These forms were read by most of the people at the school, including the director who had been a disabled child himself. I found them all very understanding. Peter's history of birth trauma, forceps delivery, bed-wetting, delayed speech, temper tantrums, distractability and lack of concentration were common for the students at this school. Most of them had also gone to numerous professionals, since most parents of hyperactive children do try to find any kind of help. The school felt Peter should be tested for his learning development, knowledge and skills.

Peter had great anxiety when he went in for his battery of tests. I hoped for some magic as I waited that day while Peter was in the testing room.

> There was a gigantic wooden jigsaw puzzle in the waiting room. It became symbolic to me. I felt there had to be a way to put it together. Peter was a puzzle. There must be a way to put him together. Everything has a solution.

Peter came out after the first hour of testing and flopped on the couch next to me. After the second hour he had had enough. He ran out of the building and locked himself in my car. My usual feelings of embarrassment and hesitation followed. The director decided we would not force Peter any more that day and we could reschedule the last event which was a talk with the psychologist. I wondered if Peter could handle another psychologist since he had seen four by now in his life.

The school chose their tests especially to determine the hard-to-measure aptitudes of the children who came in. Their I.Q. was estimated since each test measured individual ability compared to the average I.Q. The tests were set up to show ability above or below the standard level. A variation of 10 points on either side was considered significant. The following tests were given:

1. Wechsler Intelligence Scale for Children
2. Peabody Picture Vocabulary Test
3. Durrell Analysis of Reading Difficulty
4. Slosson Oral Reading Test
5. Stanford Spelling Test
6. Berea Visual Motor Gestalt Test
7. Detroit Tests of Learning Aptitude

His scores on the first test were average with a few peaks in comprehension, social judgment and reasoning. He also had superior ability to abstract visually in block design. Then, when tested to abstract verbally, he went back to the average range. His lowest scores (below average) were in arithmetic and auditory input (reproducing or finding on paper something you had to hear first.) The second test required him to point to the one picture out of four which best described a word being spoken. It was to determine if stored information exceeded expressed knowledge. His score placed him in the superior classification, indicating his underachievement was not a problem of intelligence. He was observed to have disorganization in his sentence structure and word finding problems were exhibited. His reproduction of the alphabet was labored and took over a minute to write. He also had difficulty in distinguishing upper and lower case letters. On the third test, he tested at a 3.5 grade level but his ability to comprehend what he had read varied from fair to excellent. Peter's errors in reading consisted of omitting words, guessing at them or adding suffixes. The fourth test showed similar difficulties, such as guessing a word from its first letter. During the reading tests, he was particularly fidgety and was unable to sustain his attention span. On the fifth test he was able to spell only on a 1.7 grade level. The sixth involved reproducing designs after seeing them for a set time, and he showed distortions in directionality, detail and integration. He exhibited poor serial memory, inconsistent attention, and inability to follow directions on the last test.

Peter was evaluated to exhibit underachievement, low self-esteem and insecurity. His intellectual potential was felt to be bright average to superior. They also felt his perceptual problems were in auditory and visual areas. He needed both hearing and seeing input to learn more effectively. It was felt his lag in some language skills would eventually begin to hamper him, especially in language and math, and his frustrations and anxieties would probably become greater. They said that if he did not get help soon his behavioral reactions would increase.

We had found an answer, and some help, but there was no magic. Now, I was convinced there was a solution for the puzzle of Peter, but Peter himself did not know this. He had by now been rejected, teased, and criticized, plus he saw himself as an incapable and unintelligent child. He had given up and there was nothing anyone could do to make him happy. Although Jeff had turned Peter over to me to worry about, he had supported my decision to put Peter in this school for learning disabilities. I didn't see any way out of my relationship with Jeff since he had one method and life style and Peter and I had another.

Peter left the school he was in that November and was transferred to this special school. He was to be a day student. His reaction was one of anger, more frustration and almost bitterness as he seemed to believe now that he really was dumb. His sessions of block throwing, paper ripping and destruction became so bad that in two weeks it was decided he should become a resident at the school.

For some reason I felt mostly responsible for Peter's failure and the heartache I felt to lose him was unbearable. The first few weeks he suffered from homesickness and sadness. At first, he felt rejected and betrayed, but then he began to feel sorry for some of the things he had done. He mentioned at one point he was sorry about making me take him to see all the train crossing signals. The fact that Peter even expressed a feeling was progress. He told one of the boys at the school about his mother and how nice she was. He felt guilty for how he had been so frustrated with me. Our separation from Peter was good for the rest of the family. Jeff felt relief and Eric was no longer intimidated. Apparently the tension and nervousness we all felt when Peter was around, wasn't good for Peter either and this showed in his changing attitude.

At the school his learning disabilities were individualized and he was placed at the level that he had tested at. It was a hard year for Peter. He was forced to begin to take care of his own clothes, and be more responsible. My feeling of wanting to protect him was still very strong but I could see he now had to go through some pain. The staff at the school was young and full of energy and mostly men. Since he could come home only one weekend every two weeks, he became part of their structured routine. I watched how they approached these kids and saw what they expected of them. Even though the new life was good for him, he was never happy there that year and lived in fear he would have to live at the school again the next fall.

However, while Peter did quite well that fall, Jeff again lost his job. He found one that he wanted back in Connecticut and was to begin at the end of January. I knew inside I couldn't go. I finally decided to go to a therapist myself. I wanted desperately to begin to function again since I knew Peter could not cope with a mother who was negative. He needed a strong parent who could establish a pattern for him to follow. His father was strong and stern and expected precision from all of us, but the way he presented this frightened even me. Besides, I could never live up to his perfection, nor could Peter.

> The hardest thing I learned was I could not help him until I changed myself. I unwittingly expected later to fail so some of this was obviously caused by me.

I will never forget my first visit with the therapist. He seemed to be the type of person I could like, soft spoken, warm and unassuming. After discussing my history and pressing problems, I had to tell him I didn't want to move with my husband. His response was that I didn't have to do anything I didn't want to do, and it seemed to relieve me of a kind of obligation to satisfy everyone but myself. That first day was only the beginning of months of learning why I had acted the way I did. The fact I didn't care about myself lead to some of the reasons Peter had such low self-esteem. The next months offered many problems since my husband did move away, and for the first time in Peter's life I had to show him I could handle myself.

Peter was living at home again and going to bed was hell. I would put one child to bed and the other would get up. Peter would drag Eric out of bed or hold on to him to try to keep him awake and moving with him. I used self restraint and found myself to be quite strong. Peter would lash out at me and often throw things, but we survived. I was really determined to try to handle him. One night it was ten o'clock and the violence was so great that I finally decided to call the child psychologist to help with Peter as soon as possible. Peter had learning problems but I decided the emotional ones needed to be solved first. Through all these years Peter had said two things: that I didn't love him and that no one ever listened to what he said. I was now beginning to listen to what he was saying. That, in essence, was what the psychologist was to do also. And now, I was going to have to raise my self-esteem in order for Peter to raise his.

By spring, things had improved and I surely was trying hard to change. Peter was to go to the public school half days and the other school half days. I'm sure it was very hard for him to come into a class of strange kids in April of the school year. He complained about the fact that he was missing science and fun subjects in the public school. Besides, their approach to math was different and this frustration went on for weeks before he could verbalize it. He still could not tell anyone his internal thoughts. Thus the frustration would build and either explode or he would take it out on his brother. I was told I had to establish limits for him as these hyperactive children need to know exactly what is expected of them. Whenever he missed school that spring, I was told I would have to make sure that he stayed in bed. On one of those days, he threw my watch down the drain spout, flooded the toilet, and broke a camera. But I held fast to my conviction that he had to stay in bed if he stayed home from school. One day the next week he didn't feel well enough to go to school. I explained he would have to stay in bed again and intended to keep my word. After an hour, I asked him if it was really worth it not to be able to play with the kids after school that day, and he agreed to go to school. I have never had a going-to-school problem since that day.

I now believe in what I want for him. Peter doesn't like his own bad behavior. The fact that he developed control over others gave him a power he didn't know how to cope with. He is just a child.

I was functioning as a single parent and had a dogged determination to accomplish all I could. The summer that year went better. Peter went away to camp, which wasn't hard for him since he had the experience of living away from home already. There were several other trips, one with his father on a boat and another to see his cousins at a lake. He had a good summer and could talk about some fun times. He missed his father and loves him very much, but the tension has diminished, the expectation for him is becoming more realistic and he even said to me once, *"I like you!"* I knew we were making progress when I heard that.

Peter is ten and a half now and shows steady improvement in self-esteem. It has become so noticeable that Peter's special help teacher said, "He isn't the same boy we saw last year. He comes in depressed sometimes but is now able to tell us what is bothering him. He tries harder on his work and has a more positive attitude." I hadn't expected the changes to show so soon at school.

He still has some difficulty in getting to sleep and it isn't always early, but I don't get nervous about it and just keep expecting him to accomplish it and realize that it is difficult for him. He now babysits that same little brother that he was beating on six month ago. The television was removed to the attic for the year to reinforce my belief that its distractibility is particularly harmful. He never had the discipline to turn it off by himself. The fights we have had over the TV couldn't have been worth what he got from it. I rarely shout at him but do expect certain things. If he resists, I quickly reassess my goal and see if I can let him do it later. He can express his not wanting to do it, but I go right ahead and expect him to do the task. He will usually do it and *then* I'm happy.

At times I have to listen to certain comments. "Someone will have to love you a lot to want to marry you with that tremendous tail behind you." (Tail is my kids, of course, and one in particular). My brother told my parents with honest concern: "I won't be surprised if he burns the house down." Other friends cannot believe I have such a commitment to reverse the environment of my children and often think I should get away. This does mean a lot to me and I have to stick to this conviction.

> I have discovered, now that I am a single parent, that I was indeed organized and had the right ideas for Peter. My inability to accomplish things was bound up in the complex relationship between my husband, a child and myself.

A SUMMARY OF STEPS AND IDEAS I DERIVED FOR PETER'S DAILY LIFE

The first thing parents must do is to examine their own heredity. Many early learning difficulties such as the ability to spell, to remember directions someone gives you orally, or turning numbers around after you have read them (dialing a phone number) are disabilities we have learned to compensate for as adults. Disorganization, the inability to put things in order physically, or organizing our work may be other areas that we may have a struggle to do, even today. The parent may find he gets frustrated in trying to complete certain tasks that are difficult for him because of poor fine motor control, or poor eye and hand coordination. It might be threading a needle, nailing a nail, or trying to play baseball. The parent may not understand this. He may want his child not to fail as he had, and thus will push and criticize him for the child's inability. The reasons that the parent and child have a difficulty often are never examined, and only the resentment and hostility arising from the inability to do the task appear. Their heredity may pass the trait on to their child and unless the parent can realize his own failings and compensations, will he try and correct them and help the child to learn how to cope. Understanding will be the most essential part of a loving and working household. The following areas I found to be very important to change as I concentrated on my positive efforts:

1. Disorganization—The child is by his own nature disorganized. His distractibility will make it difficult for him to complete a task. It is desirable and necessary for the child to live in an orderly environment. It seems better for the parent to either organize or help the child become organized. This may consist of room organization of books, toys, and clothes. Also time organization will bring the child some awareness of how to schedule his work and play. If a task is to be done, the child benefits greatly from knowing ahead of time that he has to perform a task. He seems to prepare himself mentally for it. If the goal is to clean up his room, the parent and child may work on the job together letting the child give his ideas where he wants things placed. Make sure the task is completed and the child will feel pleased and you will feel you have accomplished a major undertaking. The result of keeping order is that the child becomes used to the order and it becomes an environmental standard. It will help in his ability to organize his personal things, as well as his time.

2. The need this kind of child has to be loved is even greater because of his negativistic behavior. I needed to be told by the last child psychologist that Peter doesn't like the power he feels over people in his manipulation and destructive trends. This type of child needs to feel you are more in control than he is. He needs to realize from you that you know he is good. He has the normal feelings of fear, rejection (which by now he has plenty of), and the need for love and tactile contact. Peter resented all my attempts to love him as a baby for his own reasons but he did not, as I interpreted, resent me. He loved me as any child would love a parent. He wanted love and affection back from us but what he got was guilt from our frequent rejections. It is a little harder to love a child who continually embarrasses you. This negativism that persisted through Peter's early years was in part due to my lack of positiveness. I found I had some hurt feelings from when I was a child. My parents had been very negative to me. If I wanted to try something new, they would say, "You don't want to do that. It will be too difficult," or, "Don't you want to be like Jane. Who would you like to be like?" With this type of criticism, I

began to doubt not only what I wanted to do but whether I could indeed do it. My parents wanted me to be happy but they also wanted me to stay around them so they wouldn't lose me. They almost accomplished this and I was very frightened to leave them. I realized, as a mother, I was doing the same thing to Peter. I criticized him for all he couldn't do, compared him to other children who seemed to be brighter, and made him feel incapable. I therefore had to absolutely change my approach to Peter and learn a new way of letting him know that I knew he could do a task or achieve a goal that I had thought through as being possible for him.

> There is a goal that can be accomplished every day. It will make you — the parent — feel great because he has done something, and he will be happy because HE CAN DO SOMETHING TO PLEASE YOU!

3. This child will take on an authority role in some cases and talk like a dictator, but strangely enough, he cannot take his own medicine back. He will be hurt and resentful. The parent authority role needs firmness, but it must be presented in a friendly manner with a joke now and then. Peter said we never kidded or joked. He was right, we were too serious. A teasing way of saying "Oh, I know you hate to do this," or, "Really, is that so," when he refuses to do something mean a great deal. The main thing is to not give up the goal if you are sure it is a realistic expectation. It takes time, thought and planning to decide what goals you want to try with your child. I decided to concentrate with Peter on his table manners. I wanted him to learn to say, "will you please do--!", not, "get me the---." I also wanted him to ask to be excused from the table after meal time. I hope to be able to teach him how to converse at meal time and not be distracted by his brother. I will have to separate the two boys for meals if they cannot do this while sitting together. Eric can be a cause of Peter's

distractedness when Peter is trying to concentrate and be attentive. I have other goals for Peter but I have to plan when and where to start working toward them. The most important thing I must remind myself is not to start too many new things at once and, if Peter reacts negatively, I have overloaded him.

> Your standards for this child should not lessen just because of his problems, but the approach has to be quite different from the normal functioning child.

4. Diet—As the evidence becomes more apparent that hyperactive children could be affected by additives or certain dyes in food, I have made a conscious effort to avoid anything with preservatives, and stress non-processed foods. I found initially he had eaten a starchy diet with too many snack foods. First, I had to change this pattern and then gradually change Peter. I did nothing overnight as the sudden changes would have caused too much of a shock. This is where my strategy would come in and I would plan to do a little more everyday, with a long range goal in mind. The better diet also helped his constipation problems. Peter will now eat a piece of fruit at bedtime rather than something starchy.

5. I found that exposing him to higher concepts than he could learn through the orderly pattern of school, was good for him. There is a lot of energy to be channeled and the more I can channel this into interests in the world about him, the more excitement I hope will come out of the whole idea of learning. Today, at age ten, Peter cannot write a paper on tropical fish or gerbils but he could tell you orally; he has a wealth of information in his head. The idea that he is a part of a bigger world than his own little town may also help him to feel his expectations don't have to live and die here. There will be other places and hopes. The technique of quickly diverting attention when sibling problems arise is the only solution I can see. It takes a mental catalogue of ideas and a favorite book or two to catch the overactive mind and channel it back into calmness. I

have found good records can catch their minds for longer periods and are good for increasing listening skills. The records I found best are ones with good stories or poetry. The rhythm of poetry can be very enjoyable. Poetry by John Ciardi or David McCord is written especially for children. I have a record of each of them reading their own poetry. Some classical music has been recorded with a narrative and Peter always seems to enjoy this type of record. He will never put a record of this type on by himself, but when it is bedtime and he is restless, I will put one on and it usually has a quieting effect. He likes to repeatedly listen to the same record if he is enjoying it. I am not surprised to discover that he has memorized most of the record. I like to read more sophisticated children's books to him. He likes *Alice in Wonderland, Winnie the Pooh, The Little Prince.* The fact that he enjoys them so much is very encouraging to me. He must not be a dull child. He will learn to play the piano a little and I will try him on the cello. He is over ten now so he is better able to manipulate his fingers. I will not try to push him but expect him to try for a minute or two a day to learn a little more. I am amazed he retains all he has learned over the past four years in music. The higher I keep *my* goals and believe in Peter, the greater I find my reward.

I have a goal that is my legacy for Peter: to teach him to use his own resources to his fullest ability and to love himself. Without the latter, he will never succeed.

THE DISADVANTAGED CHILD

Comments by a Special Needs Teacher

A true picture of the problem of the hyperactive child would not be complete without some comments regarding disadvantaged children. The comments here are based on interviews with professional people involved in special programs for hyperactive children. These are their opinions.

Hyperactivity is best defined as a symptom of underlying developmental disorder. It is rarely an isolated problem, but instead related to a wide variety of possible neurological, emotional, or other disorders of the body as a whole. For example, hyperactivity may result from brain damage or central nervous system dysfunction, a metabolic disorder such as hypoglycemia (low blood sugar), or thyroid imbalance, and may also be a behavioral indicator of emotional disturbance. The best treatment program requires an adequate medical evaluation in order to determine the basis for a behavior disorder. If medication is appropriate, that decision rests necessarily upon determining the specific reasons for the hyperactive behavior.

Once a comprehensive medical assessment has been completed it is essential to perform a psychological evaluation of the child. The psychologist will determine the child's level of academic functioning and assess any emotional disturbance that may be present. This evaluation is critical in planning a treatment program for the hyperactive child. It is important to fully understand his intellectual potential as well as identifying any specific learning disabilities that he may have so that academic expectations for him are accurate. If emotional immaturity or instability is present, this will need to be considered in working through the behavior problems. The psychologist will assume responsibility for devising appropriate behavior modification therapy as well as suggesting alternative school programs or possible classroom modifications. The psychologist will probably recommend family counseling in order to help parents achieve an adequate adjustment to the child's disability and to learn how to effectively work with the behavior problems.

The hyperactive child clearly needs a team of professionals working together to remediate his problems. This may mean years of special therapy, special education, and continued medical consultation. This also means a lot of money and maximal understanding provided by the child's family. Unfortunately, many developmentally delayed children do not have such resources available.

At best the hyperactive child has tremendous problems to overcome. If these problems are compounded by environmental deprivation and parental neglect or abuse, the child has a very poor chance of reaching his developmental potential. For example, how can a child reach his potential in a home where the father slaps him against the wall, the mother burns him with cigarettes, or where he is tied to a bedpost and starved? Such conditions prevail! Amidst this, an impoverished family simply does not have the financial resources to secure all of the supportive therapy that the child may need. The home itself may offer very little emotional and intellectual enrichment. At the far extreme of such situations, the child may be severely punished (as mentioned previously) for behavior beyond his control or he may experience brutal rejection by his parents. The hyperactive child has little self-control to begin with, and confronted with a constantly frustrating or threatening environment will learn to defend himself either by withdrawing or fighting back. If a pattern of severe withdrawal exists, the child is no longer in touch with his world which means that the learning process and socialization will be seriously retarded. Conversely, if he becomes hostile and aggressive, which often happens, significant delinquent behavior patterns can be expected.

Clearly, any child in a deprived environment is going to suffer, but a highly vulnerable child will suffer even more. Developmentally delayed children lack the flexibility and coping capacity that normal children possess; they are almost like lame ducks or targets for abuse. A hurt child needs all of the nurturant mending that we can provide; denied, he slowly bleeds to death. There is hope for the developmentally delayed child whose parents can understand and accept his handicap and who are able to meet his needs. There is little hope for a child with special needs who must struggle simply to survive.

What can be done about such problems? The magnitude of this problem is overwhelming; there are no simple answers. These children cannot be ignored or forgotten; they belong to our society and they are our responsibility. The only hope for them is in our commitment to strive to provide a more adequate delivery of mental health services for all children who need that. We need more free clinics and intervention programs. We must comprehend the necessity in making long term treatment available for all disadvantaged children in every community in this country. These programs are expensive and the burden must be shouldered by our society. It will require much more state and federal funding which will mean substantial support from legislators and taxpayers. Our children are our most important national resource; no sacrifice seems too great when one thinks of what it is like to be a handicapped child waiting for help. Lipservice will not change it for these children, but caring enough to provide treatment facilities for them can make the difference between their being chronically maladjusted human beings and their becoming effective and independent members of our society. These children are struggling to grow beyond their handicaps; we should at least meet them halfway.

AFTERWORD

In the forward to the book I mentioned that I had learned a lot, not only by having to write about my own experiences in raising a hyperactive child, but most of all through the stories of the other parents. I thought I would close the book by discussing the things which were most revealing to me. Again, these are strictly my opinions, and not those of a professional.

1. *Guilt and anger are common in most parents of hyperactive children.* This is especially true in the early stages of a child's development. Having these feelings is a "normal" part of being the parent of a hyperactive child. Why? It is quite typical with this type of child to "never get anything back." One's love for this type of child is "forever giving," and "rarely getting." Even the most mature adult needs some amount of love in return, but in the case of a child who is rarely happy, persistent with demands, and never content more than a few minutes, it is difficult to see the "payoff" for bringing that child into the world. The payoffs are there, but it takes a psychological turnaround to find them and put them into the proper perspective. Remember, some part of this child's negative behavior is probably due to some physical-neurological impairment. Your proper managing can increase or decrease the negative behavior, but it is not all the result of incorrect actions on your part.

2. *A hyperactive child in the home typically causes strain between parents.* You do not have a bad marriage because you

have strains over a child. My wife and I have come to some kind of an "agreement" with one another. We know we are going to have disagreements when we are involved with the children. That works for us. We wear two hats, one with the kids, and another when alone. A very common strain results from fathers who deny the existence of the problem. He blames the behavior of the child on the mother. Both parents have to accept the fact that the child has a problem, one which is not caused by either parent. Also, the father *cannot* leave this problem for the mother to handle. The stories provided strong evidence that families who have a positive grasp on the problem, are those in which the father is *actively* involved in working with the mother on the problem.

3. *Physical signs of hyperactivity.* I became aware through reading these stories that many hyperactive children have some type of difficulties with fine and gross motor skills, some type of stomach trouble (colic, diarrhea, constipation), some sleeping problems, and to quote someone I once heard in a meeting, "over-response to incidental stimuli." For example, the child is in a room with some amount of noise and a train whistle blows outside (the incidental stimuli) and he says "What is that noise?" Probably, no one else heard the whistle.

4. *Most friends and family outside the home will not understand the problem.* This is simply something you had better prepare yourself for. They are *not* going to understand! You will commonly hear comments like, "She is OK!," "He is just being a child," or "Everything will work itself out." Put a dollar in a piggy bank each time it happens. Then take the money, have a big night out, and forget you ever heard the comments. I think part of this is understandable when you reconsider the doctor's introduction to this book where he defines a hyperactive child as an "exaggerated normal child." Friends and family, outside the home, usually see the child for just short periods of time. The child may seem "bratty" to them, but because they can leave the problem, it is easy for them to underplay it and brush it off. The reality is that they do not have to live with the problem continuously from the birth of the child.

5. *Helping the child is very much a matter of building his self-esteem.* This type of child needs to be successful; he needs

the right kind of love (love is not enough, but it helps the most). What is needed is an "unqualified loving" which takes the form of "love support for short term goals." This can be exemplified by ignoring petty behaviors (which might be negatively reinforced with a normal child) and heaping love and praise on any kind of positive behaviors. This takes work and patience, for the positive behaviors may be long in coming. Look for smaller things to reinforce. For instance, if the child behaves well in the car on the way to the store, reward him verbally or with a piece of candy. Redefine your goals for the child. Instead of expecting him to stick with an activity for an hour, be pleased if he makes it 10 or 15 minutes. This type of child needs limits carefully and consistently defined. He must have structure in which to form desirable behaviors.

6. *Maintain constant medical, neurological, and psychological evaluation.* These children can change in their learning abilities, their medical needs, and their physical diagnoses.

7. *What about medication?* Again, I hesitate to say anything about this for fear of playing doctor. Remember, this is *my* opinion. I recently attended a conference on learning disabilities. Each time a speaker implied avoiding medication a subgroup of the audience (maybe one-third) applauded. It was almost as if they were begging to be told not to use medication. To me the answer lies in two sentences the doctor wrote in the introduction. They affected me more than anything I have read, so much so that they bear repeating: "Some medications have also proved helpful in helping increase the child's awareness and attention span. These drugs do nothing to control behavior in themselves or make a child good or bad; they are not a substitute for loving acceptance, special methods teaching, firm limits and direction, one-on-one attention and parent-parent, parent-teacher, and parent-doctor communications in a truthful, trustful relationship." The greatest error my wife and I went through was thinking a pill will make a hyperactive child a "normal" child. That is not the purpose. The purpose is to increase awareness and attention span. The same doctor told me that different drugs have different effects on these children and they are hard to predict. Expect finding the right medication to be a trial and error process. Work closely with your doctor.

8. *What about counseling?* From the stories, it is not too difficult to surmise that there are indeed professional people who are not very helpful when it comes to dealing with hyperactive children. Too many of the parents had frustrating experiences, though most eventually found help. Which is not to say that are not many, many professional people who can help you (I think there are more all the time). What I am trying to say is that just picking someone at random, may not solve your problems. You may need to try several people, before finding the one that is the most helpful to you. For us, the best counselor was a professional who herself had a hyperactive child, but such a person may be hard to find.

9. *Beware of gimmicks.* This point did not come from the stories, but just from two experiences I have had. Two 'cures' will be given fictitious descriptions, but the stories that surround them are true. The first occurred at the same learning disability conference I mentioned earlier. A speaker was explaining this great method, known fictitiously as "The Corncob Flip-flop Reflex." It was found in most children with learning disabilities. If it could be cured, their troubles would be over. The speaker went on to say that while he could not divulge the cure, if you would only come down to his clinic and pay $1800, you could have the cure. It might indeed have been a cure. I have no evidence either way, but an expensive "secret" like that sure made me wary. The second incident was about an article which I read in a newspaper explaining how, fictitiously, "tying the child's big toes together would cure hyperactivity." I mentioned this to the director of the school for special children which my son attends. She told me she dreaded to go to school the next day, fearing to see how many children would have their big toes tied together. Again, I have no knowledge as to whether this might have worked. My point is talk to your doctor, ask him whether there is sound medical evidence supporting a possible aid to your child. Have medical studies been made which replicate the results? Proceed cautiously and hold on to your common sense. Remember, we as parents of hyperactive children are so desperate for help that we become easy prey to fast answers. For us we have never come to complete peace with our problem, but each day, each week, each year, things get better.

GLOSSARY

Ataxic: Pronounced muscle underdevelopment and generalized weakness—a staggering gait.

Benadryl® : An antihistamine used in allergic reactions and as a sedative for hyperactive children.

Breech birth: A birth in which the buttocks are presented first in contrast to a normal birth in which the head comes first.

Cerebral Palsy: Brain damage involving the cerebellum and/or related areas controlling motor function or coordinated movement.

Cesarean section: An incision in the abdominal wall and the uterine wall for the purpose of delivering a baby.

Cylert® : A stimulant used to increase the awareness of children.

Diamox® : A diuretic used to reduce fluid retention and, frequently in epileptic patients, to increase drug absorption.

Dilantin® : A seizure medication (anticonvulsant) used sometimes with hyperactive children. Its main use is to treat epilepsy.

Developmental delay: A term associated with a child who is significantly behind the developmental norms for that child's chronological age. Developments such as social, speech, gross motor skills and fine motor skills are affected.

Dexadrine® : A stimulant used to increase the awareness of hyperactive children.

EEG: See *electroencephalograph.*

Electroencephalograph: The tracing made by a device which detects and records brain waves. Used to discern stable or unstable patients. Different seizure disorders have different patterns for various areas of the brain.

Episiotomy: An incision made at the opening of the vagina to facilitate birth.

Fine motor skills: Skills associated with the use of small muscles, such as in the fingers. For example, threading string, pinching, handling a pencil, and cutting with scissors.

Flaccid hemiplegia: Impaired muscle control (floppy) on one side.

Gross motor skills: Skills associated with the use of large muscles. For example, skills such as jumping, hopping, running, skipping, bike riding, and swimming.

Hemiplegia: Paralysis of one side of the body.

Hyperactive Syndrome: An exaggerated normal child. A child with one or more of the personality types; docile, easy-to-please, passive, hard-to-please, easily-channeled behavior, aggressive, search and destroy behavior.

Hyperkinesis: Abnormal sensitivity to external stimuli resulting in inappropriate behavioral responses and overactivity.

Hyperventilation: Very deep rapid breathing.

Hypertonicity: Increased muscle and nerve tone (reflex).

Hypotonicity: Decreased muscle and nerve tone (reflex).

Large motor skills: See *gross motor skills.*

MBD: See *minimal brain dysfunction.*

Mellaril® : A combination tranquilizer, antidepressant, and mild stimulant used with hyperactive children.

Minimal brain dysfunction: Abnormality associated with brain damage that would not be detectable if an autopsy were performed. Simply stated, if the brain were cut open, no abnormality could be discerned.

Motor skills: See *fine motor skills* and *gross motor skills.*

Phenobarbitol: A sedative.

Phenergan® : Antihistamine used for food allergies, control of nausea, and as a sedative.

Rh Factor: Antigen antibody reaction between mother's serum and baby's red blood cells which destroys baby's red blood cells.

Ritalin® : A stimulant used to increase the awareness of hyperactive children.

Roseola: A viral eruption often mimicking measles often accompanied by a high fever.

Small motor skills: See *fine motor skills.*

Spastic hemiplegia: Impaired muscle control (of the stiff variety) on one side.

Tonicity: Muscle tone and reflex potential.

® Refers to brand name as opposed to generic name of drug.